Simple Fitness and Nutrition Guide for Over 60+ Active Agers.

HB Mostafa.

Contents

Welcome to a Healthier, Happier You: The Importance of Fitness and Nutrition Over 60

Welcome to a Healthier, Happier You: The Importance of Fitness and Nutrition Over 60

Turning 60 is often seen as a milestone, a time to reflect on the past and contemplate the future. It's also a natural point to re-evaluate your priorities and make changes for a healthier, happier you. Two of the most powerful tools you have for achieving this are fitness and nutrition.

Why is this so important?

As we age, our bodies naturally experience changes. Our metabolism slows down, muscle mass decreases, and bone density weakens. These changes can lead to increased risk of chronic diseases like heart disease, diabetes, and osteoporosis. However, the good news is that you have the power to counteract these effects and improve your overall well-being through regular exercise and healthy eating.

Fitness:

- Boosts energy levels: Regular physical activity increases your heart rate and oxygen flow, giving you a natural energy boost and reducing fatigue.

- Improves muscle strength and flexibility: Maintaining muscle mass not only helps you look good but also improves your balance, coordination, and reduces the risk of falls.

Flexibility exercises keep your joints limber and pain-free, allowing you to move with ease and grace.

- Strengthens bones: Weight-bearing exercises like walking, dancing, and strength training help maintain bone density, reducing the risk of osteoporosis and fractures.

- Improves mood and reduces stress: Exercise releases endorphins, the body's natural feel-good chemicals, that elevate your mood and combat stress and anxiety.

- Promotes better sleep: Regular physical activity can help you fall asleep faster and sleep more soundly, leading to improved cognitive function and overall well-being.

Nutrition:

- Provides essential nutrients: Eating a balanced diet rich in fruits, vegetables, whole grains, and lean protein ensures your body gets the vitamins, minerals, and other nutrients it needs to function optimally.

- Maintains a healthy weight: Choosing nutrient-dense foods and practicing mindful eating helps you manage your weight, reducing the risk of obesity-related health problems.

- Reduces chronic disease risk: A healthy diet can help lower your blood pressure, cholesterol, and blood sugar levels, reducing the risk of heart disease, stroke, and diabetes.

- Improves cognitive function: Eating brain-boosting foods like berries, leafy greens, and fatty fish can help maintain memory, focus, and cognitive abilities as you age.

- Increases energy levels: Nourishing your body with the right foods provides sustained energy throughout the day, preventing fatigue and sluggishness.

It's never too late to start!

Whether you've been active all your life or haven't exercised in years, incorporating fitness and healthy eating into your routine at any age can have a significant impact on your health and happiness. Remember, even small changes can make a big difference. Start by adding a short walk to your day, swapping sugary drinks for water, or incorporating a serving of vegetables into your meals.

This book is your guide to making these positive changes. We'll explore easy workout routines you can do at home or outdoors, delicious and nutritious recipes that are perfect for any meal, and helpful tips for staying motivated and on track. We'll also share inspiring stories of people over 60 who have transformed their lives through fitness and healthy eating, proving that it's never too late to embrace a healthier, happier you.

So, get ready to embark on a journey of self-discovery and empowerment. Let's turn 60 into a springboard for a vibrant, fulfilling future, one step, one bite, at a time.

Remember, you are the architect of your own health and happiness. Take charge, embrace the power of fitness and nutrition, and unlock a healthier, happier you!

In the next chapter, we'll dive deeper into why this book is your perfect roadmap to well-being, and explore the myths and misconceptions surrounding fitness and nutrition after 60.

Why This Book? Your Roadmap to Well-Being

Why This Book? Your Roadmap to Well-Being After 60

Turning 60 can feel like a significant milestone, a time to reflect on the past and contemplate the future. It's often seen as a point of transition, the end of one chapter and the beginning of another. But instead of approaching it with apprehension or resignation, imagine turning 60 as an opportunity. An opportunity to reawaken your potential, reclaim your health, and embark on a journey of self-discovery and empowerment.

This book is your guide on that journey. It's your roadmap to well-being, specifically crafted for you, the vibrant individual over 60 who knows that the best is yet to come.

Why is this book different?

Because it understands that your journey is unique. Unlike generic fitness guides or cookbooks, this book recognizes the challenges and opportunities that come with aging. It acknowledges that you may have aches and pains you didn't have before, that your metabolism might have slowed down, and that your energy levels might fluctuate. But it also celebrates your resilience, your wisdom, and your unwavering spirit.

Think of this book as your trusty companion:

- It's not a drill sergeant yelling at you to do more push-ups. It's a friendly coach, cheering you on and celebrating every small victory.

- It's not a rigid meal plan that leaves you feeling deprived. It's a culinary artist, offering a delightful buffet of flavorful, healthy recipes that nourish your body and soul.

- It's not a lecture on what you're "supposed" to do. It's a supportive friend, listening to your concerns and tailoring its advice to your specific needs and preferences.

Here's what you can expect:

- Easy-to-follow workout routines: No fancy equipment needed, just simple exercises you can do at home or outdoors, at your own pace and comfort level.

- Delicious and nutritious recipes: Forget bland, boring meals! We'll show you how to create mouthwatering dishes that are good for you and tantalize your taste buds.

- Motivational tips and tricks: Staying on track can be tough, but we'll share clever strategies to overcome challenges and celebrate milestones.

- Inspiring stories: Meet real people over 60 who have transformed their lives through fitness and healthy eating. Their stories will prove that age is just a number, and you can achieve anything you set your mind to.

- Practical advice for everyday life: From managing stress to improving sleep, we'll cover all the bases to help you feel your best every day.

But most importantly, this book is about finding joy in the process. It's about rediscovering the pleasure of movement, the fun of trying new things, and the satisfaction of nourishing your body with delicious, healthy food. It's about reframing aging as an adventure, not a sentence.

Because let's face it, 60 is not the end. It's a new beginning, a chance to rewrite your story with health, happiness, and vitality as your guiding lights. This book is your compass, your map, your cheering squad – everything you need to embark on the most incredible journey of your life: the journey to your healthiest, happiest you.

So, are you ready? Get ready to turn the page, embrace the adventure, and discover the boundless potential that lies within you. Your roadmap to well-being awaits!

In the next chapter, we'll break down the myths and misconceptions surrounding fitness and nutrition after 60. We'll debunk the excuses and empower you to approach your health with confidence and clarity.

Remember, you've got this! And this book is here to guide you every step of the way.

Dispelling Myths and Embracing Your Unique Body

Dispelling Myths and Embracing Your Unique Body: Your Key to Success Over 60

Turning 60 is often accompanied by a chorus of whispers, both internal and external, about what your body can and cannot do. These whispers morph into myths, limitations masquerading as truths, holding you back from embracing the vibrant life that awaits you. Let's bust some of these myths and pave the way for a joyous, empowered journey towards well-being.

Myth #1: You're too old to exercise.
Age is just a number. Forget the image of frail individuals struggling through grueling workouts. Fitness comes in all shapes and sizes, and finding yours is key. You can walk, dance, swim, cycle, do yoga, or even garden – the possibilities are endless. Start small, listen to your body, and celebrate every step, every bend, every beat of your heart that gets you moving.

Myth #2: Strength training is for the young.
Building muscle isn't just about bulging biceps. It's about maintaining bone density, preventing falls, and improving your daily activities. Light weights, resistance bands, or even your own bodyweight can be your tools. Embrace gentle strength training, notice the newfound power in your everyday movements, and feel the confidence radiate from within.

Myth #3: Your metabolism is broken, so weight loss is impossible.

While your metabolism might slow down slightly with age, it's not a death sentence. Focus on building muscle, which naturally boosts your metabolic rate. Choose nutrient-dense foods over processed options, and move your body regularly. Celebrate smaller portions, mindful eating, and gradual, sustainable weight loss that leaves you feeling energized and empowered.

Myth #4: You have to eat bland, restrictive food to be healthy. Flavor and nutrition can happily coexist! Healthy eating isn't about deprivation; it's about abundance. Explore the vibrant world of fruits, vegetables, whole grains, and lean protein. Discover flavorful herbs and spices that dance on your tongue. Rediscover the joy of cooking, of creating delicious meals that nourish your body and soul. Celebrate variety, experimentation, and the satisfaction of knowing you're fueling your body with the good stuff.

Myth #5: You have to push through pain to see results. Pain is your body's way of communicating. Listen to it! Modify exercises, take rest days, and adjust your routines to suit your unique needs. You can still challenge yourself, but always within a safe and comfortable range. Embrace the gentle strength you cultivate by respecting your body's limits, and celebrate the progress that comes from mindful movement.

Myth #6: You can't change your health habits at this age. It's never too late to learn, grow, and evolve. Your brain is remarkably adaptable, and new habits can be formed at any age. Start small, celebrate daily wins, and don't be afraid to stumble – just get back up and keep going. Embrace the journey of self-discovery, the joy of trying new things, and the power of small steps that lead to lasting change.

Remember, your body is not an enemy to be conquered but a partner to be cherished. Embrace its quirks, celebrate its strengths, and listen to its whispers. This journey to well-being is about honoring your unique body, about finding movement and nourishment that brings you joy, and about rediscovering the potential that lies within.

In the next chapter, we'll dive deeper into the world of "Easy Workouts for Every Body," exploring gentle, effective routines that cater to your unique needs and preferences. Get ready to move, to feel the wind on your face, and to celebrate the joy of rediscovering your body's strength and resilience!

Remember, you are beautiful, you are powerful, and you are capable of amazing things. Embrace your unique body, dispel the myths, and embark on a journey of well-being that will leave you feeling your best at any age. I'm here to cheer you on every step of the way!

Part 1: Easy Workouts for Every Body

Chapter 1: Getting Started: Overcoming Your Hesitations and Setting Realistic Goals

Identifying Your "Why": What Motivates You to Move?

Identifying Your "Why": What Motivates You to Move?

Stepping onto the journey towards a healthier, happier you might feel daunting, especially when confronted with the blank canvas of a workout routine. Before diving headfirst into exercises and meal plans, let's take a moment to identify your "why." What ignites your inner spark, whispers encouragement when your resolve falters, and propels you forward on this exciting adventure?

Finding your "why" is about uncovering the intrinsic motivators that drive you, not the external pressures or societal expectations. Forget the fleeting desire to fit into a particular dress size or impress someone at the gym. Dig deeper, explore your authentic desires.

Perhaps your "why" whispers:

- Strengthening your body to climb mountains again, dance with your grandchildren, or simply navigate daily life with ease.

- Boosting your energy levels to chase after adventures, embrace spontaneity, and live life to the fullest.

- Improving your sleep, leaving behind restless nights and waking up refreshed and ready to tackle the day.

- Enhancing your mood, combating stress and anxiety, and embracing life with a smile.

- Investing in your long-term health, reducing your risk of chronic diseases and ensuring you can enjoy life for years to come.

- Rediscovering the joy of movement, connecting with your body in a playful and empowering way.

- Building confidence and self-esteem, radiating positivity and inspiring others around you.

Your "why" is unique, personal, and powerful. It's the invisible thread that weaves through your journey, keeping you motivated when challenges arise. It's the fuel that ignites your determination when doubts creep in. It's the voice that whispers, "Remember why you started," when motivation wanes.

Here are some exercises to help you identify your "why":

- Imagine yourself a year from now. What does your life look and feel like? How has your relationship with your body changed? What are you doing that you couldn't before?

- Close your eyes and visualize movement. What kind of activity brings you joy? Is it the rhythm of a walk, the grace of a yoga pose, the exhilaration of a dance, or the strength of a push-up?

- Make a list of things you love. How can fitness enhance your enjoyment of those activities? Can it give you more energy for travel, improve your focus for creative pursuits, or boost your stamina for long hikes?

- Talk to people who inspire you with their healthy lifestyles. What motivates them? What lessons can you learn from their journeys?

Once you've identified your "why," write it down! Stick it on your fridge, your mirror, your phone – keep it visible as a constant reminder of what fuels your fire. Let it be your personal mantra, your guiding light when the path ahead seems murky.

Remember, your "why" is not set in stone. It can evolve, grow, and transform alongside you. Embrace its fluidity, and be open to discovering new reasons to move, to nourish, and to celebrate your vibrant life.

In the next section, we'll explore the art of setting realistic goals, tailored to your unique "why" and capabilities. We'll learn to translate your aspirations into achievable steps, celebrating every milestone along the way. With a clear "why" and measurable goals, your journey towards well-being becomes an adventure filled with purpose, joy, and lasting success.

Let your "why" be your compass, your motivation, your unwavering flame. Start your engines, dear reader, for the exciting journey towards a healthier, happier you begins now!

Assessing Your Fitness Level: Listen to Your Body

Before stepping onto the dance floor of your fitness journey, take a moment to tune into your body's rhythm. Assessing your current fitness level isn't about judgment, it's about self-awareness. It's a conversation with your body, a gentle exploration of its strengths and limitations, a map to guide you towards the perfect starting point.

Forget crash courses and extreme challenges. This is your own, personal symphony, and you get to choose the tempo. Remember, there's no "right" or "wrong" level, just your unique starting point on the path to a healthier, happier you.

Here's how to listen to your body's song:

1. Activity Recall: Take a mental stroll through your typical day. How much movement do you incorporate? Do you walk for errands, take the stairs, or spend most of your time seated? Understanding your current activity level sets the baseline for progress.

2. Cardio Check: Let's test your heart's beat. Walk briskly for 10 minutes and note your breathing and heart rate. Can you carry on a conversation comfortably? Do you feel breathless or fatigued? This quick test gives you a glimpse of your current cardiovascular endurance.

3. Strength & Flexibility: Time for a body scan! Can you easily get up and down from a chair? Hold a plank for 30 seconds? Touch your toes without straining? These simple tests offer insights into your muscle strength and flexibility.

4. Listen to Your Body's Whispers: Pay attention to any aches, pains, or limitations. This isn't about stopping you; it's about modifying your journey. If your knees protest during squats, opt for gentler leg

exercises. If your shoulder twinges during push-ups, try wall push-ups instead. Honor your body's messages, and adjust your routine accordingly.

Remember, your fitness level is not a fixed number. It's a dynamic melody, constantly evolving with you. Celebrate small improvements, listen to your body's whispers, and be kind to yourself throughout the process. Every step you take, every breath you deepen, is a note in your personal symphony of well-being.

Here are some helpful tips for assessing your fitness level:

- Consult your doctor: This is especially important if you have any chronic health conditions, pre-existing injuries, or concerns about starting a new exercise routine.

- Take an online fitness quiz: Several websites offer free quizzes that give you a basic assessment of your fitness level.

- Seek professional guidance: A certified personal trainer can provide a personalized assessment and design a workout plan tailored to your needs and goals.

Most importantly, approach this assessment with curiosity and kindness. It's not about achieving a certain level; it's about understanding your body's unique song and finding the movement that makes your heart sing. No matter your starting point, you have the potential to create a beautiful melody of health and well-being.

In the next section, we'll explore the art of setting realistic goals, aligning them with your "why" and your current fitness level. We'll learn to craft achievable milestones that celebrate progress, keep you motivated, and guide you on your personalized journey towards a vibrant, healthy you.

Remember, your body is an instrument of strength and grace. Tune into its unique song, listen to its whispers, and embark on a symphony of movement that resonates with your heart and soul.

Setting SMART Goals: Specific, Measurable, Achievable, Relevant, Time-Bound

The path to well-being is paved with intention. Without clear directions, excitement can wane and motivation can drift like autumn leaves. Enter the world of SMART goals, your trusty compass on this exciting adventure. SMART stands for Specific, Measurable, Achievable, Relevant, and Time-Bound, and here's how they'll guide you to success:

Specificity: Forget vague aspirations like "being healthier." Get laser-focused. Do you want to walk for 30 minutes three times a week? Strengthen your core with planks for two minutes a day? Choose one specific goal to tackle first.

Measurability: Numbers bring clarity. How will you know you've reached your goal? Count steps, track minutes, or note down the number of push-ups you can do. Seeing progress in tangible ways fuels your motivation and keeps you on track.

Achievability: Dream big, but keep your feet on the ground. Don't aim for a marathon if you haven't walked a mile in years. Start small, with bite-sized goals you can comfortably achieve. Gradual progress is key to staying motivated and building sustainable habits.

Relevance: Your goals should align with your "why." Is it to increase energy for playing with grandchildren? Reduce stress for better sleep? Make sure your goals resonate with your deepest desires and motivate you to keep moving forward.

Time-Bound: Procrastination is a master of disguise. Give your goals a deadline! Aim to walk for 30 minutes by the end of the week, master 10 push-ups in a month, or incorporate five servings of vegetables into your daily diet by next quarter. Having a timeframe adds urgency and keeps you accountable.

SMART goals are powerful tools. They transform vague aspirations into actionable steps, guiding you towards visible progress and lasting change. Here are some bonus tips for setting SMART goals:

- Break down larger goals into smaller, weekly or daily milestones. This makes them less daunting and easier to track.
- Celebrate your achievements, no matter how small. Every step counts, and acknowledging your progress fuels your motivation.
- Be flexible and adjust your goals as needed. Life throws curveballs, so adapt your plan with kindness and self-compassion.
- Don't be afraid to seek support. Share your goals with friends, family, or a fitness buddy for encouragement and accountability.

Remember, SMART goals are not rigid chains but flexible guides. Embrace their power, use them to navigate your journey, and watch as your fitness adventure unfolds with purpose, progress, and unwavering motivation.

In the next section, we'll delve into the world of building a support system – a network of encouragers, cheerleaders, and fellow travelers who walk alongside you on the path to well-being. Remember, with clear goals and a supportive network, your journey towards a healthier, happier you is bound to be filled with joy, achievement, and the thrill of exceeding your own expectations.

So, dear reader, grab your map of SMART goals, choose your first destination, and set off on your exciting adventure!

Building a Support System: Encouragement and Accountability

Building a Support System: Encouragement and Accountability on Your Journey

Embarking on a journey of well-being can feel daunting, like navigating a dense forest with only a compass to guide you. But remember, you're not alone. Building a support system – a network of encouragement, accountability, and shared enthusiasm – can be the difference between a solitary trek and a vibrant, joyful dance along the path.

Think of your support system as your cheerleading squad, your pit crew, your fellow adventurers. They are the ones who high-five you at milestones, dust you off after stumbles, and remind you of the breathtaking view that awaits at the summit.

So, who can be part of your support system?

- Family and friends: Share your goals, your excitement, and your challenges. Their genuine encouragement and understanding can be a powerful motivator.

- Workout buddy: Find someone who shares your fitness goals or simply enjoys moving. Exercising together adds a dose of fun and accountability, making workouts feel less like chores.

- Online communities: Join online forums or groups dedicated to fitness and healthy living. Connect with people who understand your journey and offer valuable tips, inspiration, and virtual high-fives.

- Personal trainer or coach: If you need more personalized guidance, consider working with a professional. They can design a tailored workout plan, answer your questions, and provide expert support every step of the way.

- Accountability apps and tools: Utilize technology to your advantage! Many apps track your progress, remind you of workouts, and even connect you with virtual fitness communities.

Here are some ways to leverage your support system:

- Share your goals and milestones. Let your cheerleaders know what you're aiming for, and celebrate your victories together.

- Schedule workout dates. Having a friend to meet for a walk, bike ride, or gym session makes exercise more enjoyable and keeps you committed.

- Seek advice and support during challenges. We all face setbacks. Reach out to your support system for encouragement, tips, and a reminder of your "why."

- Motivate others in return. Sharing your journey and offering support to others strengthens your own commitment and creates a positive ripple effect.

- Celebrate big and small wins together. Every step counts! Acknowledge your progress, however minor it may seem, and revel in the joy of moving closer to your goals.

Building a strong support system takes time and effort, but the rewards are invaluable. With a network of encouragement and accountability cheering you on, your journey towards well-being becomes a shared adventure, filled with laughter, camaraderie, and the shared joy of achieving incredible things together.

Remember, you are not alone on this path. Lean on your support system, let their strength fuel your own, and celebrate every step as you navigate the vibrant forest of well-being with a smile on your face and a song in your heart.

In the next chapter, we'll delve into the wonderful world of "Easy Workouts for Every Body," exploring gentle, effective routines that cater to your unique needs and preferences. Get ready to move, to feel the wind on your face, and to discover the boundless joy of rediscovering your body's strength and resilience!

Remember, with your "why" as your compass, SMART goals as your map, and a supportive network cheering you on, your journey towards a healthier, happier you is destined to be an adventure filled with joy, success, and endless possibilities. Now, let's lace up our metaphorical shoes and embark on this exciting journey together!

Chapter 2: The Power of Walking: Your Everyday Ally for Fitness

Walking for Overall Health: Benefits Beyond Weight Loss

Walking for Overall Health: Benefits Beyond Weight Loss

Let's talk about walking, not just as a leisurely stroll or a way to burn a few calories, but as a powerhouse for overall health and well-being. This simple, accessible activity, enjoyed by people of all ages and abilities, unlocks a treasure chest of benefits that go far beyond the number on the scale.

Why is walking so magical? Here are just a few reasons:

- Cardiovascular Champion: Walking gets your heart pumping, strengthens your heart muscles, and improves blood flow. This translates to lower blood pressure, reduced risk of heart disease, and a boost in your overall cardiovascular health.

- Mood Master: Feeling down? Lace up your shoes! Walking releases endorphins, the body's natural feel-good chemicals, reducing stress, anxiety, and depression. It can leave you feeling refreshed, energized, and ready to tackle the day with a smile.

- Bone Builder: As we age, bone density can decrease, increasing the risk of osteoporosis. Regular walking helps maintain bone strength, improving balance, reducing the risk of falls, and keeping you active and independent for longer.

- Sleep Superhero: Struggling to catch those zzz's? Walking can be your bedtime buddy! Regular physical activity regulates your sleep patterns, leading to deeper sleep and leaving you feeling more rested and energized during the day.

- Brain Booster: Walking gets your blood flowing, not just to your legs, but also to your brain. This can improve cognitive function, memory, and focus, keeping your mind sharp and ready to tackle new challenges.

- Diabetes Defense: For those with diabetes, walking can be a powerful tool for managing blood sugar levels. It helps your body use insulin more effectively, keeping your blood sugar within a healthy range.

- Joint Joy: Gentle, low-impact walking is kind to your joints, offering a great way to stay active without added strain. It can even help manage joint pain and stiffness associated with arthritis.

- Social Magnet: Walking can be a social activity! Grab a friend or family member and enjoy a chat while you stroll. Joining a walking group can be a great way to meet new people, build connections, and stay motivated.

- Fresh Air Fix: Take your walk outdoors and breathe in the fresh air. Nature has a calming effect, reducing stress and improving your mood. Enjoy the scenery, listen to the birdsong, and reconnect with the beauty of the world around you.

Remember, every step counts! You don't need to spend hours pounding the pavement to reap the benefits of walking. Start with short walks around your neighborhood, gradually increasing the duration and intensity as you become comfortable.

Here are some tips to make your walking routine enjoyable and sustainable:

- Find a walking buddy: Sharing the experience adds fun and accountability.

- Explore different routes: Keep things interesting by trying new paths and scenery.

- Listen to music or podcasts: Make your walk an entertainment experience.

- Invest in comfortable shoes: Proper footwear makes all the difference in your comfort and enjoyment.

- Track your progress: Use a pedometer or fitness tracker to see your progress and stay motivated.

- Reward yourself: Celebrate your milestones with small treats or non-food rewards.

Walking is more than just a physical activity; it's a journey towards a healthier, happier you. It's a stress reliever, a mood booster, a social activity, and a gateway to a more vibrant life. So, lace up your shoes, step outside, and let the power of walking transform your well-being one step at a time.

In the next section, we'll explore various walking workouts you can easily incorporate into your routine, from gentle strolls to interval training. Get ready to move your body, feel the sun on your skin, and discover the joy of walking towards a healthier, happier you!

Remember, every step is a small victory, a celebration of your commitment to well-being. So, step forward with confidence, dear reader, and let the power of walking unlock the treasure chest of health and happiness that awaits you every time you lace up your shoes.

Choosing the Right Gear: Shoes, Clothes, and Accessories

Step Up Your Walk: Choosing the Right Gear for Comfort and Performance

Walking is a gift you give your body: the joy of movement, the embrace of fresh air, and the freedom to explore. But to truly unlock this gift, you need the right gear – your trusty companions on your path to well-being. Let's explore the essentials that will make your walks comfortable, safe, and enjoyable, every step of the way.

Footwear Fundamentals:

Your shoes are the foundation of your walking experience. Choose wisely! Look for:

- Support and Cushioning: Opt for shoes with good arch support and adequate cushioning, especially if you walk on hard surfaces. Gel or air-cushioned soles can absorb shock and prevent discomfort.

- Fit: Shoes should fit snugly but not tightly. Leave some wiggle room for your toes to breathe and prevent blisters. Try on shoes with the socks you'll wear for walking.

- Material: Breathable mesh or leather uppers allow your feet to air out and prevent sweating. Avoid stiff, non-breathable materials that can cause blisters.

- Traction: Consider the terrain you'll be walking on. Choose shoes with good tread for uneven surfaces or wet conditions.

Comfort Counts:

Beyond shoes, the right clothing sets the stage for a pleasant walk:

- Moisture-wicking Fabrics: Fabrics like Dri-Fit or CoolMax draw sweat away from your skin, keeping you cool and dry, especially on warm days. Avoid cotton, which absorbs moisture and can make you feel clammy.

- Layering for Adaptability: Dress in layers so you can adjust to changing temperatures. A breathable windbreaker or light jacket can be a lifesaver if the wind picks up or a sudden shower rolls in.

- Comfortable Fit: Avoid loose clothing that can chafe or snag, but also ditch constricting garments that limit your movement. Choose clothes that allow for a full range of motion.

Safety First:

Visibility is key, especially if you walk at dusk or dawn. Invest in:

- Reflective Gear: Opt for clothing with reflective elements or wear a reflective vest to be seen by motorists and cyclists.

- Sunscreen and Hat: Protect yourself from the sun's harmful rays with sunscreen and a wide-brimmed hat, especially in hot weather.

- Emergency Essentials: Be prepared for the unexpected. Carry a small bag with essentials like water, a phone, identification, and any medications you might need.

Accessorize for Enjoyment:

Some extras can enhance your walking experience:

- Hydration Pack or Water Bottle: Stay hydrated with a convenient way to carry water, especially on longer walks.

- Walking Poles: Poles can improve balance, posture, and reduce stress on your knees, particularly on hilly terrain.

- Music or Podcast Player: Tune in to your favorite tunes or podcasts to make your walk more entertaining.

- Comfortable Socks: Avoid blisters with socks made from moisture-wicking materials and avoid seams that can rub.

Remember, the right gear is an investment in your well-being. Choose quality items that fit well, serve your needs, and make your walks comfortable and enjoyable. With the right shoes, clothes, and accessories, you'll be ready to conquer any path and unlock the full potential of this powerful activity.

In the next section, we'll delve into a variety of walking workouts, from relaxing strolls to energizing interval training. Get ready to discover different ways to move your body, challenge yourself, and experience the joy of walking in all its forms. So, grab your gear, step outside, and let the adventure begin!

Remember, every walk is a step towards a healthier, happier you. Choose the gear that empowers you to move with confidence and embrace the magic of walking one comfortable, stylish step at a time.

Creating Walkable Routines: Variety and Enjoyment

Create Walkable Routines: Injecting Variety and Joy into Your Stride

Walking shouldn't feel like a monotonous trek to tick off a box. It can be a vibrant tapestry woven with variety, challenge, and most importantly, enjoyment. Let's explore ways to craft walking routines that make you want to lace up your shoes and embrace the rhythm of your feet hitting the pavement.

Variety is the Spice of Life (and Walking):

- Theme Walks: Turn your walk into a mini-adventure. Embark on a historical walk, exploring landmarks; an architectural treasure hunt, seeking unique buildings; or a nature scavenger hunt, searching for birds, flowers, or specific sights.

- Interval Power: Spice up your stroll with intervals! Alternate between brisk walking and slow walking, or even jogging and walking, to boost your heart rate and burn more calories.

- Terrain Tamers: Don't be confined to concrete! Explore trails, parks, beaches, or even your own backyard. New terrain challenges your muscles and provides fresh scenery.

- Walking Buddies: Share the joy! Walk with friends, family, or even join a walking group. Social interaction keeps you motivated and adds a dose of laughter to your journey.

- Seasonal Shifts: Embrace the changing seasons! Enjoy a brisk fall walk with the leaves crunching underfoot, a leisurely winter stroll bundled up in warm layers, a spring walk amidst blooming flowers, or a breezy summer walk by the water.

Fueling Your Fun:

- Soundtrack Strolls: Put on your favorite playlist or podcast and let the music or stories propel you forward.

- Audiobook Adventures: Get lost in a captivating audiobook while you walk. Time will fly by as you're transported to another world.

- Nature's Symphony: Tune into the sounds of nature – birdsong, rustling leaves, the babbling of a brook. Let the natural world soothe your mind and recharge your spirit.

- Mindful Steps: Turn your walk into a moving meditation. Focus on your breath, your body's sensations, and the rhythm of your steps. Be present in the moment and reap the benefits of mindfulness.

Small Steps, Big Rewards:

- Start Small, Dream Big: Begin with short, manageable walks and gradually increase duration and intensity over time. Celebrate every milestone, no matter how small.

- Track Your Progress: Use a pedometer, fitness tracker, or app to monitor your steps and distance. Seeing your progress can be a great motivator.

- Reward Yourself: Celebrate achievements with non-food rewards like a new walking outfit, a massage, or a visit to a museum.

- Listen to Your Body: Don't push yourself too hard. Take rest days, adjust your pace when needed, and listen to your body's signals.

Remember, walking is a journey, not a destination. Embrace the freedom of movement, explore new paths, and most importantly, find joy in every step. Let your walkable routines be a celebration of your body, your connection to nature, and the simple pleasure of putting one foot in front of the other.

In the next section, we'll delve into the world of "Gentle Strength Training: Building Power Without Bulk." Discover exercises you can do at home or outdoors, using your own body weight or simple equipment, to build strength, improve balance, and enhance your overall well-being. So, lace up your shoes, gather your walking spirit, and get ready to explore the endless possibilities of this delightful activity!

Remember, every walk is a step towards a healthier, happier you. Let variety and enjoyment be your compass, and create routines that make you want to walk, skip, and dance your way to well-being, one joyful step at a time.

Interval Walking: Boosting Intensity for Extra Benefits

Walking is a powerful ally in your well-being journey, offering countless benefits from improved mood to heart health. But for those seeking an extra challenge and a potential calorie-torching boost, interval walking emerges as a dynamic and effective tool.

Forget marathon sprints or gym-bound intensity. Interval walking is all about strategic bursts of higher-intensity walking interspersed with recovery periods. Think alternating brisk walking with leisurely strolling, or even jogging with walking breaks. This simple yet potent practice unlocks a treasure trove of advantages:

Turbocharged Calorie Burn: The secret sauce lies in the metabolic dance your body performs during intervals. The high-intensity bursts rev up your metabolism, pushing it to burn more calories not only during the walk but also in the afterburn – that magical window where your body keeps torching extra fuel even after you've stopped.

Cardio Kickstart: Interval walking elevates your heart rate, providing a fantastic workout for your cardiovascular system. This strengthens your heart muscle, improves blood flow, and boosts your overall lung function. Say goodbye to breathlessness on the stairs and hello to a stamina-powered you!

Strength and Power Builder: Don't be fooled by the walking label. Interval training engages various muscle groups, especially your legs, core, and glutes. The high-intensity bursts challenge your muscles, leading to increased strength and power, even without fancy equipment.

Mental Agility Booster: Interval walking isn't just a physical tune-up; it's a mental boost too! The constant transitions between intensities keep your brain sharp and adaptable, improving focus, concentration, and even overall cognitive function.

Variety and Excitement: Forget the treadmill monotony! Interval walking throws in a curveball of excitement. Play with different intervals, experiment with different terrains, and embrace the freedom of choosing your own workout landscape. No more boring routines, just a dynamic dance with your own pace and preferences.

Getting Started with Interval Walking Magic:

- Warm-up: Begin with a gentle 5-10 minute walk to prepare your body.
- Choose your intervals: Start with manageable bursts, like 30 seconds of brisk walking followed by 60 seconds of recovery pace.
- Gradually increase intensity: As you get comfortable, challenge yourself by increasing the pace or duration of your high-intensity intervals.
- Listen to your body: Don't push yourself too hard. Take rest days and adjust your intervals based on your fitness level and energy.

- Mix it up: Keep your workouts fresh by exploring different terrains, adding incline variations, or incorporating walking lunges or arm swings during the high-intensity periods.

-

Remember, interval walking is a personalized journey. There's no one-size-fits-all approach. Discover what works best for you, listen to your body, and most importantly, embrace the joy of movement.

In the next section, we'll explore the wonders of "Strength Training for Everyone: Building Power Without Bulk." Discover simple, effective exercises you can do at home or outdoors to enhance your walking experience and overall well-being. So, lace up your sneakers, crank up the intensity, and unleash the hidden power within your everyday stride!

Remember, every interval walk is a step towards a stronger, healthier you. Let your body be your playground, experiment with different rhythms, and find the groove that makes your heart sing and your muscles scream (in a good way!). The path to well-being awaits, one exhilarating interval at a time.

Chapter 3: Strength Training Made Simple: Building Stronger Muscles Over 60

Why Strength Training Matters: Bone Density, Balance, and Daily Function

Let's bust a myth: strength training isn't just for bodybuilders and gym rats. It's a powerful tool for everyone, especially for those of us over 60. No, we're not aiming for bulging biceps or Olympic lifts. We're on a mission to build a stronger, healthier, and more vibrant version of ourselves, one gentle exercise at a time.

So, why should strength training be a staple in your 60+ lifestyle? Here are just a few reasons that go beyond the number on the scale:

Building Bone Density: As we age, bone density naturally decreases, increasing the risk of osteoporosis and fractures. Strength training stimulates bone-building cells, helping to maintain and even increase bone density, making you stronger and more resistant to falls. Imagine navigating stairs with confidence, enjoying your grandchildren's playful bumps, and embracing life with the sturdy foundation of strong bones.

Enhancing Balance and Stability: Forget the fear of wobbly walks and shaky handshakes. Strength training improves balance and coordination, reducing your risk of falls and enhancing your confidence in everyday activities. Imagine gardening without fear of toppling over, confidently mastering that yoga pose, and gliding across the dance floor with newfound stability.

Boosting Daily Function: Forget struggling with heavy bags or feeling winded after climbing stairs. Strength training increases muscle strength and endurance, making daily tasks easier and more enjoyable. Imagine effortlessly lifting groceries, zipping up that tight zipper, and tackling your to-do list with newfound energy and ease.

Improving Metabolism and Body Composition: Yes, strength training can even aid in weight management, but its benefits go beyond just burning calories. It builds muscle mass, which, in turn, boosts your metabolism, helping you burn more calories even at rest. Imagine enjoying all your favorite foods without guilt, maintaining a healthy weight effortlessly, and radiating the confidence of a strong, well-toned body.

Promoting Mental Wellness and Overall Well-being: The benefits of strength training extend beyond the physical. It has been shown to decrease stress, improve mood, and enhance cognitive function. Imagine feeling invigorated, reducing anxiety, and sharpening your mind, all while building strength. Picture yourself embracing life with a smile, feeling positive and focused, and radiating the joy of a healthy mind and body in perfect harmony.

Remember, strength training is an investment in your future. It's not about chasing youth or unrealistic ideals; it's about building a stronger, more resilient, and vibrant version of yourself.

In the next section, we'll explore the "Gentle Exercises for Building Strength," showing you how simple, bodyweight exercises and light equipment can unlock a world of power and well-being, right at home or outdoors. So, ditch the fear of bulky weights and heavy lifting, and get ready to discover the strength that lies within!

Remember, every exercise counts, every repetition is a victory, and every step towards a stronger you is a celebration of life. Embrace the journey, listen to your body, and let the power of gentle strength training transform your well-being, one powerful moment at a time.

Bodyweight Exercises: No Equipment Needed, Big Results

Bodyweight Exercises: No Equipment Needed, Big Results Over 60

Forget intimidating gyms and expensive equipment! Your path to a stronger, healthier you over 60 begins right where you are, with the incredible power of your own body weight. These simple, yet effective exercises require no special tools, just you and your commitment to well-being.

Get ready to build strength, improve balance, and boost your energy with these bodyweight wonders:

Upper Body Powerhouse:

- Chair Dips: Sit on a sturdy chair, hands shoulder-width apart on the edge. Lower yourself down until your elbows bend at 90 degrees, then push back up. Start with modified dips from your knees until you build strength.

- Wall Push-ups: Stand facing a wall, arms shoulder-width apart slightly away from the wall. Lean in and bend your elbows, lowering your chest towards the wall. Push back up to finish. Modify on your knees or at an angle for gentler resistance.

- Rows: Use a sturdy table or counter to anchor yourself. Stand facing away, lean forward and grab the edge with straight arms. Pull your body towards the surface, engaging your back muscles. Repeat with controlled movements.

Lower Body Champions:

- Squats: Stand with feet shoulder-width apart, toes slightly outward. Lower yourself down as if sitting in a chair, keeping your back straight and core engaged. Push back up to finish. Modify by holding onto a chair for balance or squatting only as low as comfortable.

- Lunges: Step forward with one leg, lowering your body until both knees bend at 90 degrees. Push back up to start and repeat with the other leg. Modify by holding onto a wall or chair for balance, or shortening the stride for gentler intensity.

- Calf Raises: Stand on the balls of your feet, lift your heels off the ground, and hold for a few seconds before lowering back down. Modify by doing calf raises while holding onto a wall or chair for support.

Core Crusaders:

- Planks: Start on your forearms and toes, forming a straight line from head to heels. Engage your core and hold for as long as comfortable. Modify by starting on your knees or elbows for less intensity.

- Bird-Dogs: Start on all fours, hands shoulder-width apart and knees hip-width apart. Extend one arm and the opposite leg out straight, keeping your back flat and core engaged. Bring them back to center and repeat on the other side.

- Crunches: Lie on your back with knees bent, feet flat on the floor. Lift your upper body off the ground a few inches, engaging your abdominal muscles. Slowly lower back down and repeat. Modify by keeping your feet flat on the floor or doing smaller crunches.

Remember, listen to your body! Start with a few repetitions and gradually increase as you get stronger. Modify exercises as needed to suit your fitness level and avoid pain. Take rest days to allow your muscles to recover.

Here are some additional tips to maximize your bodyweight workouts:

- Focus on form: Proper form is key to maximizing results and preventing injury. Don't rush the movements; focus on controlled repetitions and engaging the targeted muscle groups.

- Breathe deeply: Inhale as you exert effort and exhale as you release. Proper breathing keeps you oxygenated and improves your workout efficiency.

- Make it fun: Turn your workout into a mini-dance party, challenge yourself with variations, or even involve family and friends for a fun group workout.

- Celebrate your progress: Don't get discouraged by slow starts. Focus on how you feel, acknowledge your improvements, and celebrate every milestone, big or small.

Bodyweight exercises are a gateway to a stronger, more vibrant you. No fancy equipment, no hefty price tags, just you and your commitment to well-being. Take the first step, embrace the power within, and witness the incredible transformation that unfolds with each repetition.

In the next section, we'll explore the world of "Light Equipment for Bigger Benefits," showcasing simple tools that can enhance your bodyweight workouts and add further variety to your fitness journey. Remember, every move counts, every exercise is a celebration, and with every step on this path, you're building a stronger, healthier you, one triumphant repetition at a time.

Resistance Bands: Your Portable Gym for Effective Workouts

Resistance Bands: Your Portable Gym for Effective Workouts Over 60

Move over, bulky weights and intimidating gym memberships! Your journey to greater strength and improved well-being over 60 takes a delightfully portable turn with the magic of resistance bands. These colorful loops of elastic goodness hold the power to transform any space – your living room, backyard, even a hotel room – into your own personalized gym, packed with endless training possibilities.

But why are resistance bands such game-changers for those of us over 60? Here's why:

Versatility Unbound: Unlike the fixed weight of dumbbells, resistance bands offer adjustable resistance. Choose lighter bands for gentle movements or challenge yourself with thicker ones for a more intense workout. This adaptability caters to your specific fitness level and allows you to progress at your own pace.

Gentle on Your Joints: Forget the jarring impact of heavy weights. Resistance bands provide a more fluid and low-impact form of resistance, making them kinder to your joints and reducing the risk of injury. Imagine confidently exercising without fear of aches and pains, embracing movement with peace of mind and renewed enjoyment.

Travel-Friendly Fitness: No more gym hassles or lugging around heavy equipment. Resistance bands are lightweight, compact, and easily portable, fitting neatly in your purse, luggage, or desk drawer.

Take your workout anywhere, anytime, and never miss a beat on your path to well-being.

Full-Body Fitness: Don't be fooled by their simple appearance. Resistance bands can target every muscle group in your body, from your upper body and core to your legs and glutes. With a variety of exercises and band positions, you can sculpt, tone, and strengthen your entire physique, building a well-rounded foundation for health and vitality.

Functional Movement Magic: Forget isolated bicep curls. Resistance bands excel at mimicking real-life movements, engaging multiple muscle groups simultaneously. Imagine improving your balance with side squats, enhancing your posture with rows, and strengthening your core with rotational exercises. These functional movements translate into everyday life, making you stronger and more confident in everything you do.

Getting Started with Your Band Bonanza:

Choose a variety of bands with different resistance levels based on your fitness level and workout goals. Start with lighter bands for gentler exercises and gradually progress to thicker bands as you get stronger.

Here are some simple yet effective exercises to get you started:

- Squats with Band Around Legs: Place the band just above your knees and squat as usual, feeling the resistance through your legs.

- Rows with Anchored Band: Secure the band to a doorknob or post, grab it with both hands, and pull your torso towards the anchor point, engaging your back muscles.

- Overhead Press with Band: Hold the band behind your head with both hands, palms facing forward. Press your arms overhead, extending your elbows fully.

- Plank with Band Variations: Place the band around your ankles or wrists during plank variations to add an extra challenge to your core stability.

Remember, listen to your body! Start with a few repetitions and gradually increase as you get stronger. Modify exercises as needed and take rest days to allow your muscles to recover.

Here are some additional tips to maximize your resistance band workouts:

- Get creative: Explore online resources and videos for endless exercise variations and workout routines.

- Incorporate intervals: Alternate between high-intensity band exercises and rest periods to boost your heart rate and burn more calories.

- Make it fun: Turn on your favorite music, involve a friend or family member, or create your own workout challenges to keep things engaging.

- Celebrate your progress: Don't get discouraged by slow starts. Track your improvements, acknowledge your achievements, and revel in the joy of becoming a stronger, fitter you.

Resistance bands are your passport to a world of fitness possibilities, right at your fingertips. Ditch the excuses, embrace the portability, and step into a stronger, healthier future, one colorful loop at a time.

Remember, every repetition is a victory, every move a celebration, and with each band-powered exercise, you're building a vibrant, well-being journey that extends far beyond the gym walls. So, grab your bands, find your space, and let the fitness magic begin!

Light Weights: Gradually Adding Resistance for Strength Gains

Light Weights: Unlocking a World of Strength Gains Over 60

Step aside, intimidating barbells and bulky dumbbells! Your path to greater strength and improved well-being over 60 takes a gentle yet effective turn with the magic of light weights. These trusty training tools, often dismissed as beginner equipment, hold the power to unlock a world of strength gains, improved balance, and enhanced confidence, all without the stress or strain of heavy lifting.

But why are light weights such game-changers for those of us over 60? Here's why:

Gradual Progression: Unlike bodyweight exercises or resistance bands, light weights offer the advantage of controlled, incremental increases in resistance. Start with weights you can comfortably lift for 10-12 repetitions, and gradually add heavier weights as you get stronger. This allows you to challenge yourself safely and consistently, witnessing progress with every workout.

Bone Density Boost: As we age, bone density naturally decreases, increasing the risk of fractures. Studies have shown that light weight training can stimulate bone-building cells, helping to maintain and even increase bone density, making you stronger and more resistant to falls. Imagine confidently navigating stairs, enjoying outdoor activities without fear of stumbles, and embracing life with a sturdy foundation of strong bones.

Muscle Maintenance and Development: Don't believe the myth that muscle building is reserved for the young. Light weight training helps maintain and even increase muscle mass over 60, leading to improved strength, power, and endurance. Imagine carrying groceries with ease, tackling household chores with renewed energy, and radiating the confidence of a stronger, more toned physique.

Improved Balance and Coordination: Forget the fear of wobbly walks and shaky handshakes. Light weight training, especially exercises that involve movement and coordination, can improve balance and stability, reducing your risk of falls and enhancing your confidence in everyday activities. Imagine mastering that yoga pose, gliding across the dance floor with newfound poise, and navigating bustling streets with unwavering balance.

Mental Wellness and Overall Well-being: The benefits of light weight training extend beyond the physical. It has been shown to reduce stress, improve mood, and enhance cognitive function. Imagine feeling invigorated, reducing anxiety, and sharpening your mind, all while building strength. Picture yourself embracing life with a smile, feeling positive and focused, and radiating the joy of a healthy mind and body in perfect harmony.

Getting Started with Your Light Weight Adventure:

Choose weights that you can comfortably lift for 10-12 repetitions with good form. Start with two sets of 10-12 repetitions per exercise, and gradually increase sets and repetitions as you get stronger.

Here are some simple yet effective exercises to get you started:

- Bicep Curls: Stand with feet shoulder-width apart, hold a weight in each hand, and curl your arms towards your shoulders, squeezing your biceps at the top.

- Overhead Press: Stand with feet shoulder-width apart, hold a weight in each hand overhead, then slowly lower them down to shoulder level and press back up.

- Tricep Extensions: Hold a weight in each hand overhead, then bend your elbows, lowering the weights behind your head until your forearms are parallel to the ground. Extend your arms back up to finish.

- Squats with Weights: Hold a weight in each hand at your sides, squat down as if sitting in a chair, keeping your back straight and core engaged. Push back up to finish.

Remember, listen to your body! Start with light weights and gradually increase as you get stronger. Modify exercises as needed and take rest days to allow your muscles to recover.

Here are some additional tips to maximize your light weight workouts:

- Focus on form: Proper form is key to maximizing results and preventing injury. Don't rush the movements; focus on controlled repetitions and engaging the targeted muscle groups.

- Breathe deeply: Inhale as you exert effort and exhale as you release. Proper breathing keeps you oxygenated and improves your workout efficiency.

- Make it fun: Turn on your favorite music, involve a friend or family member, or create your own workout challenges to keep things engaging.

- Celebrate your progress: Don't get discouraged by slow starts. Track your improvements, acknowledge your achievements, and celebrate every milestone, big or small.

Light weights are your stepping stones to a world of strength and empowerment over 60. Ditch the fear of heavy metal, embrace the controlled progression, and witness the incredible transformation that unfolds with each gentle lift. Remember, every repetition is a victory, every set a celebration, and with each light weight conquest, you're building a stronger, more vibrant you, one empowering workout at a time. So, grab your weights, find your space, and embark on a journey where progress comes in measured doses and every lift adds up to a healthier, happier you!

Chapter 4: Low-Impact Exercise Options: Gentle on Your Joints, Big on Results

Swimming: A Full-Body Workout with Minimal Impact

Dive into Wellness: Swimming – A Full-Body Workout with Minimal Impact

Forget the jarring thrum of treadmills and the bone-jarring impact of high-intensity workouts. Your path to well-being takes a refreshing, low-impact turn with the magic of swimming. Immerse yourself in a world of gentle resistance, full-body conditioning, and buoyant joy, all while taking exceptional care of your precious joints.

Why is swimming the aquatic answer to your fitness prayers over 60? Here's the deep dive:

- Joint-Friendly Oasis: Unlike land-based activities that exert stress on your knees, hips, and spine, swimming offers the perfect sanctuary for your joints. The water's buoyancy takes the weight off your body, allowing you to move freely and exercise without fear of pain or injury. Imagine gliding through the water, feeling your muscles engage without a hint of ache, and rediscovering the joy of uninhibited movement.

- Cardio Champion: Don't be fooled by the serene glide. Swimming is a fantastic cardiovascular workout, engaging your heart, lungs, and circulation with every stroke. Whether you choose a leisurely freestyle or a vigorous breaststroke, your heart will be pumping, your blood flowing, and your energy levels soaring. Picture tackling daily activities with renewed vigor, enjoying walks without getting winded, and radiating the vitality of a well-conditioned heart.

- Full-Body Fitness Factory: Ditch the isolation exercises that target specific muscle groups. Swimming is a full-body workout, engaging your arms, legs, core, and back with every stroke and kick. Imagine sculpting lean muscle, improving your posture, and building core strength – all while enjoying the refreshing embrace of the pool.

- Mental Wellness Oasis: Beyond the physical benefits, swimming offers a haven for your mental well-being. The rhythmic strokes, the soothing water, and the focus on breath combine to create a natural stress reliever and mood booster. Imagine leaving your worries at the pool's edge, feeling calm and invigorated after each swim, and carrying that serenity into your daily life.

- Social Splash Pad: Swimming isn't just a solitary pursuit. Join a water aerobics class, socialize with fellow pool enthusiasts, or even challenge your grandkids to a playful race. The social aspect adds a layer of fun and motivation, making your workouts enjoyable and enriching. Imagine laughter echoing through the pool, forging new friendships, and building a supportive community around your aquatic pursuit.

Getting Started with Your Splashing Success:

Begin with gentle laps, focusing on proper form and controlled movements. Choose strokes that feel comfortable, like freestyle or backstroke, and gradually increase distance and intensity as you get stronger.

Here are some low-impact water exercises to add variety to your routine:

- Water Walking: Take a stroll in the shallow end, engaging your legs and core as you walk against the water's resistance.

- Arm Circles: Rotate your arms in wide circles, forward and backward, targeting your shoulders and upper back muscles.

- Aqua Jogging: Jog in place in the deep end, keeping your feet off the bottom and utilizing the water's resistance for a lower-impact cardio workout.

- Aquatic Stretches: Hold gentle stretches, like leg extensions and backbends, using the water's support to deepen your stretches without strain.

Remember, listen to your body! Start slowly, take rest days, and modify exercises as needed. Don't hesitate to seek guidance from a water aerobics instructor or swim coach for personalized advice and technique improvement.

Here are some additional tips for maximizing your swimming workouts:

- Invest in a swimsuit that fits well and supports your body.

- Warm up before entering the water and cool down with gentle stretches afterward.

- Hydrate before, during, and after your swim.

- Make it fun! Explore different strokes, play water games, or listen to your favorite music while underwater.

- Celebrate your progress! Track your swimming distance, lap times, or simply the joy you feel in the water.

Swimming is more than just an exercise; it's a gateway to a vibrant, well-being journey over 60. Dive into the refreshing embrace of the water, rediscover the joy of movement, and witness the incredible transformation that unfolds with each stroke. Remember, every lap is a victory, every dive a celebration, and with each joyful splash, you're building a stronger, healthier, and happier you. So, grab your swimsuit, find your pool, and plunge into a world of aquatic wellness that redefines fitness and rekindles the joy of movement, one refreshing dip at a time!

Yoga: Flexibility, Balance, and Inner Peace

Unroll Your Mat, Unwind Your Mind: Yoga – A Pathway to Flexibility, Balance, and Inner Peace Over 60

Forget the intimidating downward dogs and gravity-defying headstands. Your path to well-being over 60 takes a gentle, mindful turn with the magic of yoga. Unroll your mat, step onto a journey of inner exploration, and discover a world of enhanced flexibility, improved balance, and profound inner peace, all without the strain or stress of high-impact exercise.

Why is yoga the perfect antidote to the stiffness and worries of life over 60? Here's the mindful pose:

- Joint-Friendly Bliss: Unlike activities that jolt your joints, yoga offers a safe haven for your body. The focus on slow, controlled movements and stretching postures protects your precious joints, allowing you to move with mindful awareness and build strength without fear of injury. Imagine bending with ease, reaching for high shelves with comfort, and rediscovering the joyful freedom of supple joints.

- Posture Powerhouse: Forget the slouch and the hunch. Yoga's emphasis on alignment and core engagement helps you improve your posture, leading to a taller, more confident stance. Imagine standing tall with unwavering presence, navigating crowds with ease, and radiating the newfound grace of a well-balanced body.

- Flexibility Fountain: Age doesn't have to mean stiffness. Yoga's gentle stretches and poses help you improve your flexibility, increasing your range of motion and reducing aches and pains. Imagine touching your toes without breaking a sweat, climbing stairs with agility, and embracing the delightful freedom of a limber body.

- Balance Booster: Forget the fear of falls and wobbly strides. Yoga's focus on balance poses and core engagement improves your stability and coordination, reducing your risk of falls and enhancing your confidence in everyday activities. Imagine navigating uneven terrain with newfound steadiness, mastering challenging yoga poses with grace, and radiating the stability of a well-anchored mind and body.

- Stress-Melting Oasis: Life can be a whirlwind, but yoga offers a refuge. The combination of breathwork, meditation, and mindful movement creates a powerful stress-reduction tool, calming your mind, easing anxiety, and promoting inner peace. Imagine leaving your worries at the edge of your mat, feeling rejuvenated after each practice, and radiating the serenity of a calm and clear mind.

Getting Started on Your Mindful Journey:

Begin with gentle poses on the floor, focusing on proper alignment and controlled movements. Choose beginner-friendly routines or join a chair yoga class if kneeling or floor poses feel challenging.

Here are some basic poses to get you started:

- Mountain Pose (Tadasana): Stand tall with your feet shoulder-width apart, arms at your sides, and spine elongated. Engage your core and gently raise your gaze.

- Tree Pose (Vrksasana): Stand on one leg, balancing your other foot on your shin or inner thigh. Engage your core and maintain a steady gaze.

- Cat-Cow Pose (Marjaryasana-Bitilasana): On all fours, arch your back as you inhale (cow pose) and round your back as you exhale (cat pose).

- Child's Pose (Balasana): Kneel with your toes together and sit back on your heels. Rest your forehead on the mat and breathe deeply.

Remember, listen to your body! Modify poses as needed, take rest days, and avoid pushing yourself to pain. Don't be afraid to use props like blocks or straps to support your practice.

Here are some additional tips for maximizing your yoga journey:

- Find a style that suits you, whether it's gentle Hatha yoga, restorative yoga, or chair yoga.

- Practice regularly, even if it's just for a few minutes each day.

- Focus on your breath and connect your movements to your breath.

- Make it fun! Turn on calming music, light candles, or practice outdoors in nature.

- Celebrate your progress! Don't compare yourself to others; focus on your own journey and enjoy the feeling of being present in your body and mind.

Yoga is more than just exercise; it's a transformative journey for your body, mind, and spirit. Unroll your mat, breathe deeply, and step onto a path of enhanced flexibility, improved balance, and profound inner peace. Remember, every pose is a victory, every breath a celebration, and with each mindful movement, you're building a stronger, calmer, and more vibrant you. So, find your center, find your breath, and unroll the magic of yoga, one graceful pose at a time!

Pilates: Core Strength and Body Control

Cultivate Core Control, Sculpt a Stronger You: Pilates – Your Key to Inner Strength Over 60

Forget bulging biceps and intimidating gym machines. Your path to well-being over 60 takes a precise, controlled turn with the magic of Pilates. This dynamic yet gentle exercise method, far from just mat exercises and stretchy bands, unlocks a world of core strength, improved posture, and refined body control, all without the strain or impact of high-intensity workouts.

Why is Pilates the perfect sculptor for a stronger, more confident you over 60? Here's the power pose explanation:

- Core Champion: Forget the dreaded backaches and wobbly balance. Pilates places its emphasis on strengthening your core muscles, your body's powerhouse. As your core stabilizes, you'll experience improved posture, reduced back pain, and enhanced balance, leading to a confident stride and everyday ease. Imagine lifting groceries without strain, navigating uneven terrain with grace, and radiating the strength of a well-supported core.

- Posture Perfectionist: Slouching takes a backseat, thanks to Pilates' focus on alignment and body awareness. You'll learn to lengthen your spine, engage your muscles strategically, and move with intention, resulting in a taller, more graceful posture that commands attention and boosts confidence. Imagine standing tall in any crowd, mastering poses with unwavering presence, and radiating the elegance of a perfectly aligned body.

- Joint-Friendly Finesse: Unlike activities that jolt your joints, Pilates' focus on controlled movements and mindful transitions protects your precious joints. You'll build strength and flexibility without the risk of injury, rediscovering the joy of uninhibited movement and embracing a pain-free path to well-being. Imagine bending easily to tie your shoes, reaching high shelves with comfort, and enjoying the delightful freedom of a well-oiled body.

- Sculpting Powerhouse: Don't be fooled by the seemingly gentle poses. Pilates engages multiple muscle groups simultaneously, leading to improved muscle tone, increased definition, and a more sculpted physique. Imagine feeling stronger in everyday activities, mastering challenging poses with finesse, and radiating the confidence of a body that moves with precision and power.

- Mind-Body Magic: Pilates isn't just about physical exercise; it's a mind-body connection odyssey. The focus on breathwork, concentration, and mindful movement creates a powerful stress-reduction tool, calming your mind, easing anxiety, and promoting inner peace. Imagine leaving your worries at the studio door, feeling rejuvenated after each session, and radiating the serenity of a calm and connected mind and body.

Getting Started on Your Pilates Path:

Begin with basic mat exercises, focusing on proper form and controlled movements. Choose beginner-friendly routines or join a class specifically designed for over 60s. Pilates equipment like reformers and chairs can be incorporated later as you progress.

Here are some basic exercises to get you started:

- Pelvic Tilts: Lie on your back with knees bent and feet flat on the floor. Tilt your pelvis inward (tuck your tailbone) and then outward, engaging your core muscles.

- Spinal Rolls: Lie on your back with arms at your sides. Gently roll your upper body off the mat, one vertebra at a time, and then slowly roll back down.

- Single-Leg Bridge: Lie on your back with knees bent and feet flat on the floor. Lift one leg up, keeping your hips level, and engage your core and gluteus muscles. Repeat with the other leg.

- Plank: Start on all fours, then extend your legs back into a push-up position with your elbows bent at 90 degrees. Engage your core and hold for as long as comfortable.

Remember, listen to your body! Modify exercises as needed, take rest days, and avoid pushing yourself to pain. Don't hesitate to seek guidance from a certified Pilates instructor for personalized advice and technique improvement.

Here are some additional tips for maximizing your Pilates journey:

- Find a qualified instructor who can tailor the program to your needs and fitness level.

- Practice regularly, even if it's just for a few minutes each day.

- Focus on your breath and connect your movements to your breath.

- Make it fun! Put on upbeat music, create a calming atmosphere, or practice with a friend.

- Celebrate your progress! Don't compare yourself to others; focus on your own journey and enjoy the feeling of control and strength you cultivate with each exercise.

Pilates is more than just an exercise; it's a transformative journey for your body, mind, and spirit. Unroll your mat, breathe deeply, and embark on a path of core strength, refined posture, and empowered movement. Remember, every pose is a victory, every breath a celebration, and with each controlled movement

Tai Chi: Graceful Movements for Mind and Body Harmony

Unfurl Your Inner Grace: Tai Chi – Movement Poetry for Mind and Body Harmony over 60

Forget the jarring thrum of treadmills and the intimidating clang of barbells. Your path to well-being over 60 takes a serene, flowing turn with the magic of Tai Chi. Imagine transforming your workout into a graceful dance, weaving together gentle movements, deep breaths, and focused awareness. Welcome to a world where strength and flexibility blossom through slow, mindful movements, and inner peace becomes a tangible reward for each deliberate step.

Why is Tai Chi the perfect elixir for a vibrant, well-balanced you over 60? Here's the harmonious breakdown:

- Joint-Cherishing Choreography: Unlike activities that jolt your joints, Tai Chi's fluid, low-impact movements protect your precious bone and cartilage. Each step, each turn, is an act of joint-soothing, allowing you to move with mindful awareness and rediscover the joy of uninhibited movement without aches or pains. Imagine navigating stairs with ease, reaching high shelves without a wince, and rediscovering the delightful freedom of a pain-free body.

- Balance Blossoming: Forget the fear of wobbly strides and unsteady footing. Tai Chi's focus on balance and weight shifting improves your stability and coordination, reducing your risk of falls and enhancing your confidence in everyday activities. Imagine gliding across uneven terrain with newfound steadiness, mastering challenging postures with unwavering presence, and radiating the grace of a well-anchored mind and body.

- Strength in Stillness: Don't be fooled by the seemingly gentle pace. Tai Chi engages multiple muscle groups, subtly building strength and improving flexibility. As you flow through graceful postures, you'll experience increased muscle tone, better range of motion, and a stronger, more defined physique. Imagine lifting groceries with renewed ease, mastering challenging poses with precision, and radiating the quiet power of a body nurtured from within.

- Stress-Melting Meditation: Life can be a whirlwind, but Tai Chi offers a sanctuary. The synchronized movements, deep breaths, and focused awareness create a powerful stress-reduction tool, calming your mind, easing anxiety, and promoting inner peace. Imagine leaving your worries at the edge of the practice space, feeling rejuvenated after each session, and radiating the serenity of a calm and clear mind.

- Mind-Body Symphony: Tai Chi isn't just about physical exercise; it's a mind-body connection odyssey. The focus on mindfulness, breathwork, and intentionality creates a harmonious connection between your thoughts, emotions, and movements, leading to a deeper sense of self-awareness and well-being. Imagine finding tranquility in each step, experiencing the joy of being present in the moment, and radiating the harmony of a body and mind in perfect sync.

Getting Started on Your Flowing Journey:

Begin with basic postures, focusing on proper form and mindful transitions. Choose beginner-friendly routines or join a class specifically designed for over 60s. Tai Chi requires no special equipment, so you can practice anywhere, anytime – your living room, a park bench, even amidst nature's embrace.

Here are some basic movements to get you started:

- Opening the Arms: Stand with feet shoulder-width apart, arms at your sides. Slowly raise your arms out to the sides, palms facing down, then back down, feeling the stretch in your chest and shoulders.

- Wild Goose Qigong: Stand with feet hip-width apart, knees slightly bent. Shift your weight to one leg, raise the other leg slightly behind you, and reach your arms forward, then repeat on the other side.

- Embrace the Tree: Stand with feet together, arms at your sides. Slowly raise your arms overhead, palms together, and imagine your arms becoming branches reaching towards the sun.

- Turn Your Waist: Stand with feet shoulder-width apart, hands on your hips. Gently rotate your torso from side to side, focusing on engaging your core muscles.

Remember, listen to your body! Modify movements as needed, take rest days, and avoid pushing yourself to pain. Don't hesitate to seek guidance from a certified Tai Chi instructor for personalized advice and technique improvement.

Here are some additional tips for maximizing your Tai Chi journey:

- Find a style that suits you, whether it's gentle Tai Chi Chuan or more energetic Yang Style.

- Practice regularly, even if it's just for a few minutes each day.

- Focus on your breath and connect your movements to your breath.

- Make it fun! Practice outdoors in nature, listen to calming music, or create a serene atmosphere in your practice space.

- Celebrate your progress! Don't compare yourself to others; focus on your own journey and enjoy the feeling of inner peace and harmony you cultivate with each mindful movement.

Tai Chi is more than just an exercise; it's a transformative journey for your body, mind, and spirit. Unfurl your inner grace, flow through each deliberate step, and witness the incredible transformation that unfolds with each mindful movement. Remember, every turn is a victory, every breath a celebration, and with each graceful posture, you're building a stronger, calmer, and more vibrant you. So, find your quiet corner, breathe deeply, and embark on a path of flowing movement, inner peace, and harmonious well-being. Let Tai Chi become your dance, your meditation, your symphony of strength and serenity, one flowing step at a time.

Beyond the physical benefits, Tai Chi can also have a profound impact on your mental and emotional well-being. Studies have shown that regular practice can:

- Reduce stress and anxiety: The slow, rhythmic movements and focused breathing of Tai Chi create a sense of calmness and relaxation, helping to quiet the mind and ease worry.

- Improve mood and reduce depression: The release of endorphins during exercise, combined with the sense of accomplishment and well-being after a practice session, can contribute to a more positive outlook and uplift your mood.

- Enhance cognitive function: Tai Chi requires focus and concentration, which can help to improve memory, attention, and overall cognitive function.

- Promote better sleep: The calming effects of Tai Chi can help you fall asleep faster and sleep more soundly, leading to improved energy levels and overall well-being.

In addition to these individual benefits, Tai Chi can also foster a sense of community and connection. Joining a Tai Chi class can be a way to meet new people, socialize, and share the experience of this meditative practice with others.

As you embark on your Tai Chi journey, remember to:

- Embrace the process: The beauty of Tai Chi is in the journey, not the destination. Focus on enjoying the movements and feeling the connection between your body and mind.

- Be patient: Learning Tai Chi takes time and practice. Don't get discouraged if you don't master all the movements right away. Just keep practicing and you will gradually improve.

- Listen to your body: Modify the movements as needed to suit your own abilities and limitations. It's important to avoid pain and injury.

- Make it your own: There are many different styles of Tai Chi. Find one that you enjoy and that fits your needs.

- Have fun! Tai Chi should be a enjoyable experience. So, relax, smile, and flow with the movements.

With dedication and practice, Tai Chi can become a lifelong companion on your path to well-being. It can help you build strength, improve balance, reduce stress, and find inner peace. So, unroll your mat, breathe deeply, and let the gentle art of Tai Chi guide you towards a vibrant, well-balanced life, one graceful movement at a time.

Chapter 5: Staying Motivated and Making Exercise a Habit

Finding the Fun: Activities You Enjoy Make Exercise Sustainable

Find Your Fit, Spark Your Flame: Making Exercise a Joyful Habit with Activities You Love

Forget the treadmill torture and forced gym visits. Ditch the guilt trips and the "no pain, no gain" mantras. The path to lasting fitness over 60 takes a delightful turn with the magic of finding activities you genuinely enjoy. Imagine, not dread, that pre-workout buzz. Picture smiles, not sweat-gripped grimaces, during your exercise adventure. Welcome to the world where motivation thrives on joy, and consistency blossoms from passion, not pressure.

Why does embracing activities you love hold the key to unlocking a sustainable exercise habit? Here's the joyful breakdown:

- Intrinsic Motivation Unleashed: Forget external pressures and fleeting trends. When you choose activities that spark your inner fire, intrinsic motivation takes the wheel. You exercise because you want to, not because you have to. The joy of dancing, the thrill of exploring nature, the satisfaction of mastering a new skill – these intrinsic motivators propel you forward, fueling consistent action without the need for willpower or self-criticism.

- Engagement Transforms Effort: Exercise morphs from a dreaded chore into a playful exploration. Whether it's the rhythm of the Zumba beat, the camaraderie of a hiking group, or the challenge of conquering a new climb, your senses are engaged, your mind is present, and the effort feels effortless. Time flies, goals become achievements, and exercise ceases to be a box to tick but a vibrant thread woven into the tapestry of your life.

- Variety Spices Up the Journey: No more one-size-fits-all monotony. Embracing a spectrum of activities keeps your mind and body stimulated, preventing boredom and plateaus. You can dance one day, swim the next, and join a book club walk the day after. Variety becomes your secret weapon, ensuring long-term engagement and preventing the dreaded exercise rut.

- Social Butterflies Take Flight: Forget solitary confinement on the treadmill. Choose activities that allow you to connect with like-minded souls, be it a tennis partner, a dance class filled with friendly faces, or a hiking group exploring hidden trails. The social aspect adds a layer of fun and support, boosting motivation, accountability, and the joy of shared experiences.

- Confidence Soars on Wings of Progress: As you master new skills, conquer challenges, and witness your own physical and mental transformation, your confidence takes flight. You feel empowered, capable, and proud of your accomplishments. This surge of confidence spills over into other areas of your life, creating a ripple effect of well-being and motivation to keep moving forward.

Finding Your Playground for Joyful Movement:

- Listen to your heart: What did you love to do as a child? Did you dance with reckless abandon? Explore the outdoors like a fearless adventurer? Reconnect with those passions and reignite the spark of joy.

- Step outside your comfort zone: Don't limit yourself to familiar territory. Try a new salsa class, join a kayaking group, or sign up for a beginner's rock climbing session. You might discover hidden talents and passions you never knew existed.

- Embrace technology: Explore fitness apps, online dance tutorials, or virtual hiking tours. The digital world offers a plethora of options to explore from the comfort of your home or discover hidden gems in your neighborhood.

- Connect with your community: Look for community centers, senior centers, or parks offering fitness classes, social groups, or organized activities. Connect with like-minded individuals and turn exercise into a vibrant social experience.

- Turn it into a family affair: Enlist your spouse, children, or grandchildren to join you in your fitness adventures. Hiking, biking, playing Frisbee in the park – shared activities not only strengthen bonds but also add a layer of fun and motivation.

Remember, there's no one-size-fits-all path to joyful movement. Don't get caught up in comparing yourself to others or chasing fad trends. The key is to listen to your inner voice, explore your passions, and find activities that spark your soul. Celebrate every step, every laugh, every accomplishment, no matter how small. Embrace the journey, not the destination, and let the joy of movement guide you toward a sustainable, vibrant, and truly fulfilling fitness habit.

Start small, dream big, and most importantly, have fun! Remember, exercise is not a punishment, it's a celebration of your amazing body and spirit. So, turn your workout into a playground, your routine into a joyful dance, and your fitness journey into a vibrant mosaic of activities you love, one playful step at a time!

Tracking Your Progress: Celebrate Milestones and Stay Inspired

Charting Your Triumphs: How Tracking Progress Fuels Motivation and Inspires Consistency

Forget the self-defeating whispers of doubt and the looming shadow of plateaus. Your path to lasting fitness over 60 takes a triumphant turn with the magic of tracking your progress. Imagine, not ignoring, the incredible milestones you achieve. Picture, not despairing over stagnant numbers, but celebrating the daily victories that pave your path to well-being. Welcome to the world where data becomes your cheerleader, where numbers transform into trophies, and every step, every challenge conquered, becomes a testament to your unwavering commitment.

Why does tracking your progress hold the key to unlocking lasting motivation and consistent action? Here's the inspiring breakdown:

- Visibility Fuels Confidence: No more hazy memories of "working out sometimes." Tracking your workouts, whether in a journal, a fitness app, or a simple calendar, brings your efforts into sharp focus. You see the tangible evidence of your dedication, the concrete steps you've taken toward your goals. This newfound visibility fuels confidence, reminding you of your strength and capabilities, and propelling you forward with renewed motivation.

- Small Victories, Big Celebrations: Forget waiting for monumental achievements to celebrate. Tracking allows you to cherish the small victories, the extra ten minutes added to your run, the mastered yoga pose, the conquered hill on your bike ride. Each checkmark, each increase in weight lifted, becomes a mini-celebration, a pat on the back that keeps you on the path and rekindles the joy of progress, no matter how incremental.

- Data Becomes Your Coach: Numbers aren't your enemy; they're your personalized roadmap. Tracking metrics like steps walked, calories burned, or distance covered allows you to identify patterns, adjust your routine, and set achievable goals. You become your own coach, empowered with data to make informed decisions and optimize your journey towards a healthier, more active you.

- Plateaus Become Stepping Stones: Remember those dreaded plateaus that used to derail your motivation? Tracking can transform them into opportunities for growth. By analyzing your data, you can identify areas for improvement, switch up your routine, or even seek guidance from a professional. Plateaus become stepping stones, pushing you to adapt, evolve, and emerge stronger than ever before.

- Accountability with a Positive Twist: Forget the guilt trips and external pressures. Tracking provides a supportive, empowering form of accountability. You're accountable to yourself, your goals, and the joy of witnessing your own progress. This positive accountability fosters a sense of ownership and pride, keeping you motivated without the need for negativity or self-criticism.

Transforming Data into Delightful Milestones:

- Choose your weapon: Find a tracking method that resonates with you. Whether it's a bullet journal filled with inspirational quotes and colorful charts, a sleek fitness app with gamified features, or a simple spreadsheet filled with your personal data – choose a tool that sparks joy and makes tracking feel like a celebration, not a chore.

- Focus on progress, not perfection: Don't get bogged down by missed workouts or occasional setbacks. Track your overall progress, celebrate the trends, and acknowledge the inevitable fluctuations that are part of any fitness journey. The key is to focus on the bigger picture, not the occasional blip on the radar.

- Share your triumphs: Don't keep your victories to yourself! Share your progress with friends, family, or even online communities. Celebrating your achievements with others amplifies the joy, strengthens your commitment, and inspires others on their own paths to well-being.

- Embrace the journey: Tracking is not about reaching a finish line; it's about enjoying the scenic route. Focus on the process, the small wins, the daily acts of self-care and movement. Let the data be your guide, not your dictator. Celebrate the journey, not just the destination, and watch your motivation blossom with every tracked step.

- Reward yourself, not punish: Ditch the self-flagellation for missed workouts. Instead, reward yourself for consistently tracking, for achieving milestones, for simply showing up and giving your best effort. This positive reinforcement system will keep you motivated, excited, and eager to continue your journey towards a healthier, happier you.

Remember, tracking your progress is not about micromanaging or obsessing over numbers. It's about celebrating your journey, acknowledging your accomplishments, and using data as a tool to empower your choices and inspire continuous movement. So, grab your journal, your app, or your whiteboard, and start charting your triumphs. Let the numbers become your cheering squad, your milestones become stepping stones, and your progress become the fuel that propels you towards a vibrant, well-being-filled future, one joyful step at a time!

Overcoming Challenges: Addressing Setbacks and Staying on Track

Bouncing Back with Grace: Embracing Setbacks and Conquering the "Blah" Days

Let's be honest, the fitness journey isn't always sunshine and rainbows. There will be days when the couch whispers sweet nothings, motivation takes a sabbatical, and the thought of another workout elicits a yawn instead of a cheer. Fear not, valiant over-60 warriors! Setbacks are a natural part of the process, and conquering them is where true resilience and lasting habits are forged. Welcome to the world where bumps become stepping stones, "blah" days morph into opportunities for growth, and every challenge overcome becomes a testament to your unwavering spirit.

Why are setbacks, instead of deterrents, our secret strength boosters? Here's the empowering breakdown:

- Redefining Failure: Ditch the negative connotations. A missed workout, a skipped session, a plateau – these are not failures, they are opportunities for introspection and adaptation. They point us towards areas for improvement, remind us of the importance of rest and self-care, and ultimately guide us to a more sustainable, personalized approach to fitness.

- Resilience Blossoms from Challenge: Every hurdle overcome, every setback bounced back from, builds psychological muscle. You learn to adapt, strategize, and come back stronger. This newfound resilience spills over into other areas of life, equipping you with the confidence to tackle challenges and navigate obstacles with unwavering grace.

- Building Sustainable Habits: Remember those rigid, all-or-nothing plans that crumbled at the first sign of a stumble? Setbacks become your teachers, nudging you towards flexible, sustainable habits. You prioritize rest and listen to your body, embrace new activities, and adjust your routine to fit your lifestyle, creating a long-term plan that thrives on adaptability, not strictness.

- Discovering Hidden Fuel: Sometimes, even the most dedicated stumble. But instead of despair, use these "blah" days as an opportunity to explore. Try a new activity, join a fun fitness class, connect with nature on a walk, or simply take a restorative yoga session. You might discover hidden passions, reignite your spark for movement, and stumble upon activities that fuel your motivation in unexpected ways.

- Celebrating Small Victories: Don't wait for monumental achievements to pat yourself on the back. Celebrate the small victories, the "I showed up today" moments, the decision to choose movement over inertia. This positive reinforcement, especially on those "blah" days, keeps you on track, reminds you of your progress, and fuels the intrinsic motivation to keep going, even when the sun isn't shining.

Equipping Yourself for Graceful Bouncing Back:

- Plan for the inevitable: Accept that setbacks are part of the journey. Build flexible routines with rest days and alternative activities, so you have options when motivation takes a nap.

- Listen to your body: Don't push through pain or exhaustion. Rest is not failure, it's recovery. Listen to your body's signals and prioritize self-care when needed.

- Embrace change: Don't get stuck in a rut. Try new activities, explore different routines, and keep your workout playlist fresh. Variety can be the antidote to boredom and reignite your enthusiasm.

- Connect with your support system: Share your challenges with friends, family, or online communities. Their encouragement and understanding can be a powerful motivator to get back on track.

- Celebrate every step: Remember, progress is not always linear. Celebrate the small victories, the consistent effort, and the journey itself. Each step, even those taken hesitantly, brings you closer to your goals.

Setbacks are not roadblocks; they are opportunities to build resilience, refine your approach, and discover a more sustainable path to well-being. So, embrace the inevitable "blah" days, learn from your stumbles, and bounce back with grace. Remember, true strength lies not in avoiding challenges, but in conquering them with unwavering spirit and a smile. Take your setbacks as stepping stones, your "blah" days as invitations to explore, and keep moving forward, one joyful, resilient step at a time!

Buddy Up! Partnering for Exercise Motivation and Social Connection

The Synergy of Sweat: Buddy Up! Partnering for Exercise Motivation and Social Connection

Forget the lonely treadmill grind and the silent pushups in your living room. Your path to lasting fitness over 60 takes a vibrant turn with the transformative power of buddying up. Imagine, not battling gym anxiety alone, but sharing smiles and high-fives with a workout partner. Picture not just sculpted muscles, but strengthened connections and a newfound social circle born from shared sweat and laughter. Welcome to the world where partnership fuels motivation, camaraderie boosts accountability, and every workout becomes a joyous celebration of movement and connection.

Why does partnering up hold the key to unlocking an irresistible, sustainable fitness habit? Here's the synergistic breakdown:

- Motivation Multiplied: Ditch the self-inflicted pep talks and the dwindling willpower. With a workout buddy, motivation becomes contagious. Seeing your partner show up, push hard, and celebrate their victories sparks your own inner fire. The shared commitment, the playful competition, the mutual encouragement – these become powerful motivators, propelling you forward even when your solo resolve might have faltered.

- Accountability with a Smile: Forget the guilt trips and internal pressure. Partnering up offers a gentle, supportive form of accountability. You nudge each other to show up, celebrate milestones, and offer a friendly reminder when motivation takes a temporary vacation. This positive accountability, devoid of negativity or judgment, keeps you on track without sacrificing the joy of movement.

- Social Fabric, Woven Through Movement: Exercise ceases to be a solitary pursuit and transforms into a shared experience. You laugh together over missed steps, commiserate over muscle fatigue, and cheer each other on through challenging poses. This social connection fosters a sense of belonging, reduces isolation, and adds a layer of joy and purpose to your fitness journey.

- Discovery Through Shared Exploration: Forget the monotony of predictable routines. With a partner, you can embark on fitness adventures together. Try a new dance class, conquer a hiking trail, or join a kayaking group. This shared exploration keeps things fresh, ignites new passions, and ensures you never get bored on your path to well-being.

- Celebration Amplified, Triumphs Shared: Forget the solitary fist pumps and silent victories. With a partner, every milestone becomes a celebration amplified. You high-five after conquering a climb, share cheers after mastering a yoga pose, and revel in each other's achievements as if they were your own. This shared joy doubles the happiness, strengthens the bond, and fuels the motivation to keep moving forward, together.

Finding Your Perfect Fitness Partner:

- Seek similar interests: Find a partner who shares your fitness goals, enjoys similar activities, and whose energy level complements yours. A harmonious partnership makes workouts more fun and ensures a shared commitment to consistency.

- Embrace diversity: Age, gender, and fitness level don't matter. The beauty of fitness partnerships lies in celebrating differences and supporting each other's journeys. Look for someone who inspires you, motivates you, and makes you feel comfortable in your own skin.

- Connect with your community: Explore community centers, senior centers, or online platforms to find potential partners. Look for fitness classes designed for pairs, join sports teams, or simply put the word out among your friends and family.

- Open communication is key: Talk openly about your goals, preferences, and limitations. Communicate when you need support, celebrate each other's victories, and offer encouragement when motivation wanes. Strong communication is the cornerstone of a thriving fitness partnership.

- Make it fun!: Choose activities you both enjoy, set playful challenges, and inject humor into your workouts. Laughter, shared experiences, and the joy of movement are the secret ingredients to keeping your partnership strong and your motivation flourishing.

Remember, partnering up is not about finding a fitness clone; it's about finding someone who complements you, challenges you, and makes your journey towards a healthier, happier you infinitely more fun and fulfilling. So, grab your friend, your spouse, or your neighbor, lace up your sneakers, and step into the vibrant world of shared sweat, contagious laughter, and a fitness journey enriched by the power of true connection. With a buddy by your side, every step becomes a celebration, every challenge a shared victory, and every workout a testament to the transformative power of movement and friendship, one joyful high-five at a time!

Part 2: Easy Healthy Recipes for Delicious Nourishment

Chapter 6: The Importance of Nutrition After 60: Fueling Your Body for Optimal Health

Understanding Your Nutritional Needs: Age-Specific Dietary Guidelines

Nourishing Your Sixty-Plus Journey: Understanding Age-Specific Dietary Guidelines

Forget the one-size-fits-all diet plans and calorie-counting anxieties. Your path to optimal health over 60 takes a personalized turn with the illuminating compass of age-specific dietary guidelines. Imagine, not deciphering complex health jargon, but embracing simple, adaptable principles that nurture your unique needs and preferences. Picture, not restrictive regulations, but a flexible framework that empowers you to make informed choices, build a vibrant plate, and fuel your body for well-being with every delicious bite. Welcome to the world where nutritional knowledge becomes your superpower, where food becomes your ally, and every meal becomes a celebration of self-care and delicious discovery.

Why are age-specific dietary guidelines your secret weapon for optimal health? Here's the nourishing breakdown:

- Understanding Your Changing Needs: As your body undergoes the natural transitions of aging, your nutritional needs subtly shift. Metabolism slows down, bone density requires attention, and maintaining muscle mass becomes increasingly important. Age-specific guidelines equip you with the knowledge to address these unique needs, ensuring you prioritize the right nutrients for sustained health and vitality.

- Personalized, Not Prescriptive: Forget rigid rules and calorie-counting restrictions. These guidelines offer a flexible framework, not a strict regimen. You have the freedom to adapt them to your individual preferences, cultural background, and health conditions, fostering a sustainable approach to well-being that honors your unique story.

- Empowering Choice, Not Deprivation: Ditch the guilt trips and deprivation tactics. Age-specific guidelines empower you to make informed choices, encouraging you to focus on nutrient-rich whole foods while still allowing for mindful indulgences. You learn to navigate food choices with confidence, prioritizing well-being without sacrificing the joy of eating.

- Fueling Your Body with Wisdom: These guidelines equip you with the knowledge to choose foods rich in the nutrients your body craves at this stage of life. You prioritize calcium for bone health, protein for muscle maintenance, and fiber for digestive regularity, ensuring your body receives the building blocks it needs to thrive.

- Preventing Future Challenges: Age-specific guidelines go beyond the immediate plate. They empower you to make choices that can help prevent chronic conditions like heart disease, diabetes, and osteoporosis. By incorporating these principles into your daily life, you invest in your long-term health and build a foundation for a vibrant, independent future.

Navigating the Nutritional Compass:

- Focus on Whole Foods: Prioritize nutrient-rich, unprocessed foods like fruits, vegetables, whole grains, lean protein, and healthy fats. These foods provide a natural abundance of vitamins, minerals, and fiber, fueling your body from the ground up.

- Befriend Calcium and Vitamin D: Calcium for strong bones and Vitamin D for efficient absorption – these dynamic duo become your bone health champions. Include calcium-rich foods like dairy, leafy greens, and tofu in your diet, and ensure adequate Vitamin D intake through sunlight exposure or supplements.

- Champion Muscle-Building Protein: Maintaining muscle mass becomes crucial over 60. Prioritize protein sources like lean meats, fish, eggs, beans, and nuts to ensure your body has the building blocks it needs for strength, mobility, and independence.

- Fiber, Your Digestive Ally: Embrace fiber-rich foods like fruits, vegetables, and whole grains to keep your digestive system healthy and regular. Adequate fiber can also help manage cholesterol and blood sugar levels, contributing to overall well-being.

- Stay Hydrated, Always: Water is your body's best friend, especially as you age. Aim for eight glasses of water daily and choose water-rich fruits and vegetables to stay hydrated and support vital bodily functions.

Remember, age-specific dietary guidelines are not a rulebook, but a roadmap. Use them to learn about your unique needs, make informed choices, and build a personalized approach to optimal health. Experiment with new flavors, explore diverse cuisines, and discover the joy of mindful eating. Celebrate your journey, not just your destination, and let your dietary choices become a delicious expression of self-care and well-being.

So, embrace the knowledge, adapt the principles, and embark on a culinary adventure fueled by informed choices and vibrant flavors. With each thoughtful bite, you nourish your body, mind, and spirit, paving the way for a joyful, vibrant, and optimally healthy journey through your sixty-plus years and beyond. Bon appétit!

Choosing Nutrient-Rich Foods: Prioritize Fruits, Vegetables, and Whole Grains

Unleash the Rainbow Power: Making Fruits, Vegetables, and Whole Grains Your Nutritional Champions

Forget bland salads and cardboard crackers. Your path to optimal health over 60 takes a vibrant, flavorful turn with the nutrient-rich bounty of fruits, vegetables, and whole grains. Imagine, not struggling with restrictive diets, but filling your plate with a kaleidoscope of colors, textures, and tastes that nurture your body and tantalize your palate. Picture, not battling nutritional deficiencies, but embracing a natural powerhouse of vitamins, minerals, and fiber that fuels your well-being with every delicious bite. Welcome to the world where food becomes medicine, your plate becomes a canvas, and every meal becomes a celebration of vibrant health and culinary discovery.

Why do fruits, vegetables, and whole grains hold the key to unlocking a thriving, well-nourished you? Here's the rainbow-hued breakdown:

- Nature's Vitamin and Mineral Bounty: Ditch the supplement overload and embrace the natural abundance. Fruits and vegetables are bursting with vitamins, minerals, and antioxidants, each color offering a unique blend of health-promoting powerhouses. From beta-carotene in carrots to vitamin C in oranges, your plate becomes a vibrant pharmacy, fueling your body and protecting it from chronic diseases.

- Fiber, Your Digestive Ally: Forget sluggish mornings and uncomfortable bloating. Whole grains and fiber-rich vegetables are champions of digestive health. They keep things moving smoothly, regulate blood sugar levels, and even contribute to lowering cholesterol, leaving you feeling energized and comfortable.

- Muscle-Loving Protein and Satiating Power: Don't underestimate the protein content of whole grains and leafy greens. These plant-based powerhouses provide essential protein for muscle maintenance and repair, along with a satisfying fiber content that keeps you feeling full and energized throughout the day.

- Brainpower Boosters: Forget the age-related memory lapses and cognitive decline. Fruits like berries and leafy green vegetables are loaded with beneficial nutrients that nourish your brain and support cognitive function. Every colorful bite becomes a small investment in mental clarity and a sharper, more vibrant mind.

- Vibrant Health Through Flavor: Ditch the bland, restrictive diets and embrace the culinary playground. Fruits, vegetables, and whole grains offer a dazzling array of flavors, textures, and colors, turning mealtimes into a joyful exploration of taste. You discover new favorites, experiment with spices and herbs, and cultivate a love for healthy eating that goes beyond mere obligation.

Building Your Vibrant Plate:

- Embrace the rainbow: Aim for a variety of colors – red, orange, yellow, green, purple – every day. Each color represents a unique blend of beneficial nutrients, ensuring you get the full spectrum of health-promoting compounds.

- Go local and seasonal: Choose fresh, locally-grown produce whenever possible. Seasonal fruits and vegetables are at their peak ripeness, bursting with flavor and nutrients. Plus, supporting local farmers adds a touch of eco-consciousness to your dietary choices.

- Make vegetables your star: Aim for half your plate to be filled with non-starchy vegetables like broccoli, spinach, kale, or peppers. These nutrient-dense powerhouses provide essential vitamins, minerals, and fiber without the extra calories.

- Befriend whole grains: Ditch the refined bread and pasta and embrace the power of whole grains like brown rice, quinoa, oats, and barley. These provide sustained energy, essential fiber, and valuable nutrients your body craves.

- Don't fear fat: Healthy fats from avocado, nuts, and seeds add flavor, satiety, and essential nutrients to your diet. Choose them in moderation and enjoy their delicious contribution to your well-being.

Remember, making fruits, vegetables, and whole grains your dietary champions is not about sacrifice, it's about celebration. Explore new recipes, get creative in the kitchen, and discover the hidden flavors and versatility of these natural health heroes. Share meals with loved ones, experiment with global cuisines, and turn mealtimes into joyful rituals of nourishment and connection.

So, open your refrigerator door, step into the vibrant world of a farmer's market, and embrace the abundance of nature's bounty. With each colorful bite, you fuel your body, nourish your mind, and paint your journey to optimal health with the vibrant strokes of delicious, well-being-infused choices. Let your plate become a masterpiece, your meals a celebration, and your health a testament to the transformative power of nature's rainbow-hued champions!

Portion Control Matters: Eating Mindfully and Avoiding Overeating

Taming the Portion Monster: Mastering Mindful Eating and Avoiding Overindulgence

Forget the guilt trips and restrictive diets. Your path to well-being over 60 takes a mindful turn with the art of portion control. Imagine, not battling oversized plates and second helpings, but cultivating a calm awareness of your body's needs and satiety cues. Picture, not succumbing to emotional eating and mindless munching, but savoring every bite with gratitude and appreciation. Welcome to the world where mindful eating becomes your superpower, your plate a balanced canvas, and every meal a conscious conversation with your body, leading to lasting well-being and joyful nourishment.

Why does mastering portion control hold the key to unlocking a healthy, vibrant you? Here's the mindful breakdown:

- Banishing the Binge Cycle: Ditch the yo-yo dieting and emotional eating sprees. Mindful eating teaches you to listen to your body's natural hunger and fullness cues, preventing overindulgence and promoting a sustainable approach to healthy eating. You develop a healthy relationship with food, free from guilt and deprivation.

- Fueling Your Body, Not Your Emotions: Forget seeking comfort in sugary treats or mindless snacking. Mindful eating helps you identify emotional triggers for overeating and empowers you to choose healthier coping mechanisms. You nourish your mind and spirit, not just your stomach, building resilience against emotional eating triggers.

- Optimizing Digestion and Energy Levels: Overeating can lead to sluggishness, bloating, and discomfort. Mindful eating promotes smaller, more frequent meals that optimize digestion, keep energy levels stable, and leave you feeling light and energized throughout the day.

- Appreciating Flavor and Texture: Ditch the mindless munching and savor every bite. Mindful eating encourages slow, deliberate eating, allowing you to truly appreciate the flavor, texture, and aroma of your food. Each meal becomes a sensory experience, enhancing your enjoyment and reducing the urge to overeat.

- Building Sustainable Habits: Mindful eating isn't a quick fix; it's a transformative shift in your relationship with food. By cultivating awareness and practicing portion control, you build sustainable habits that support your long-term health and well-being, one mindful bite at a time.

Cultivating Your Mindful Eating Journey:

- Listen to your body: Pay attention to your natural hunger and fullness cues. Eat when you're truly hungry and stop when you're comfortably satisfied, not stuffed.

- Embrace smaller plates: Downsize your dinnerware. Smaller plates visually trick your brain into feeling full with less food, promoting portion control without deprivation.

- Slow down and savor: Chew slowly and deliberately, taking the time to appreciate the flavor and texture of your food. This practice enhances digestion, increases satiety, and prevents mindless overeating.

- Minimize distractions: Turn off the TV, put away your phone, and focus on the act of eating. Avoid distractions that can cause you to lose awareness of your hunger and fullness cues.

- Plan your meals: Preparing healthy meals and snacks in advance helps you avoid impulsive choices and unhealthy options when hunger strikes. Plan portion sizes before you eat and stick to your predetermined quantities.

- Practice mindful gratitude: Be grateful for the food you have and acknowledge its role in nourishing your body. This fosters a positive relationship with food and helps you avoid emotional eating triggers.

Remember, mastering portion control is not about punishment; it's about self-compassion and gentle awareness. Don't beat yourself up over occasional stumbles; embrace them as learning opportunities and gently guide yourself back to mindful eating practices. Celebrate your progress, not just your destination, and enjoy the journey of building a healthy, sustainable relationship with food.

So, take a deep breath, slow down, and savor every bite. Listen to your body's wisdom, cultivate mindful awareness, and let portion control become your ally, not your enemy. With each conscious choice, you fuel your body with respect, nourish your mind with gratitude, and pave the way for a healthy, joyful journey towards optimal well-being, one mindful meal at a time!

Hydration for Health: Water as Your Essential Beverage

The Crystal Elixir: Embracing Water as Your Essential Beverage for Optimal Health

Forget sugary sodas and calorie-laden juices. Your path to optimal health over 60 takes a refreshingly simple turn with the crystal elixir of life – water. Imagine, not battling dehydration headaches and sluggish afternoons, but feeling vibrant and energized, every cell brimming with the essence of well-being. Picture, not reaching for sugary drinks out of habit, but quenching your thirst with the pure, delicious satisfaction of water, savoring its role as your body's vital partner in health. Welcome to the world where water becomes your superpower, your glass a crystal chalice, and every sip a celebration of internal harmony and optimal function.

Why does water hold the key to unlocking a thriving, well-hydrated you? Here's the crystal-clear breakdown:

- The Lifeblood of Every Cell: Forget fancy supplements and miracle cures. Water is the fundamental building block of life, accounting for 60% of your body weight and playing a crucial role in every vital function. From regulating temperature to transporting nutrients and flushing out toxins, water is the silent orchestra conductor, keeping your body's symphony in perfect harmony.

- Brain Booster and Mood Enhancer: Dehydration isn't just about thirst; it can impact your cognitive function and mood. Studies show even mild dehydration can lead to fatigue, confusion, and decreased alertness. Keeping your glass filled fuels your brainpower, elevates your mood, and keeps you sharp and focused throughout the day.

- Energy Unleashed: Forget the afternoon slump and caffeine dependence. Water is the fuel your body craves. Proper hydration improves blood flow, delivers oxygen to your cells, and boosts your energy levels, leaving you feeling revitalized and ready to take on the day.

- Digestive Ally and Weight Management Partner: Water keeps your digestive system running smoothly, preventing constipation and promoting regularity. Proper hydration also helps you feel full and satisfied, reducing cravings and potentially aiding in weight management efforts.

- Glowing Skin and Radiant Health: Forget expensive creams and complicated routines. Water is your natural beauty elixir. It keeps your skin plump and hydrated, flushes out toxins, and promotes a healthy, radiant glow from within. By prioritizing water, you invest in your natural beauty and let your inner health shine through.

Embracing the Crystal Elixir:

- Make water your go-to beverage: Ditch the sugary drinks and processed juices. Reach for a glass of water first thing in the morning, throughout the day, and before every meal. Carry a reusable water bottle with you to stay hydrated on the go.

- Infuse it with flavor: If plain water feels too bland, add a slice of lemon, cucumber, or berries for a natural flavor boost. Experiment with herbal teas or fruit-infused waters to keep things interesting.

- Listen to your body: Pay attention to your thirst cues. Don't wait until you're parched to reach for water. Drink proactively throughout the day to stay ahead of dehydration.

- Set reminders and track your intake: Use apps or simple timers to remind you to drink water throughout the day. Keep a water bottle with markings to track your intake and ensure you're reaching your daily goal.

- Make it fun and social: Enjoy water with friends and family. Share infused water recipes, set hydration challenges, and make water a part of your social gatherings.

Remember, embracing water is not just about quenching thirst; it's about celebrating life. Every sip is a conscious choice to nourish your body, fuel your well-being, and invest in your long-term health. So, raise your glass, savor the crystal-clear purity, and let water become your essential companion on your journey to optimal health and vibrant vitality. With each refreshing sip, you unlock a symphony of internal harmony, leaving you feeling energized, focused, and radiant from the inside out. Cheers to a life fueled by the elixir of life itself – water!

Chapter 7: Breakfast Like a Champion: Starting Your Day with Energy and Nutrition

Power-Packed Smoothies: Easy, Delicious, and Nutrient-Dense

Morning Magic in a Mug: Power-Packed Smoothies for an Energized and Nutritious Start

Forget the soggy cereal and rushed coffee mornings. Your path to a vibrant day over 60 takes a delicious, health-infused turn with the power of power-packed smoothies. Imagine, not scrambling for breakfast solutions, but blending a vibrant concoction of flavor and nutrition that fuels your body and fires up your energy engines. Picture, not settling for sugary juices or skipping breakfast altogether, but savoring a nutrient-rich smoothie that nourishes your mind, body, and spirit, setting the stage for a day of well-being and accomplishment. Welcome to the world where smoothies become your morning champions, your blender a culinary wizard, and every sip a celebration of deliciousness and vibrant health.

Why do power-packed smoothies hold the key to unlocking a winning start to your day? Here's the smoothie-rific breakdown:

- Nutritional Powerhouse in a Glass: Ditch the multivitamin overload and embrace the natural bounty. Smoothies allow you to pack in a diverse array of fruits, vegetables, whole grains, nuts, and seeds, creating a nutritional powerhouse in every sip. Vitamins, minerals, fiber, antioxidants – your smoothie becomes a personalized cocktail of well-being, tailored to your unique needs and preferences.

- Convenience Meets Flavor: Forget the rushed mornings and chaotic breakfast routines. Smoothies are a quick and easy solution, taking minutes to prepare and offering a portable, on-the-go breakfast option. No cooking, no dishes, just a delicious blend of goodness to kickstart your day.

- Digestive Delight: Ditch the heavy, greasy breakfasts that leave you feeling sluggish. Smoothies are gentle on your digestive system, providing easily absorbed nutrients and fiber to keep things moving smoothly and comfortably throughout the morning.

- Energy on Demand: Forget the dreaded afternoon slump. The nutrient-dense blend of carbohydrates, protein, and healthy fats in your smoothie provides sustained energy, keeping you focused and productive throughout the morning. No more sugar crashes or caffeine jitters, just steady, sustained fuel for your mind and body.

- Tastebud Celebration: Ditch the bland breakfasts and monotonous routines. Smoothies offer a playground for your palate. Experiment with fruits, spices, herbs, and greens, discovering new flavor combinations and culinary adventures. Each morning becomes a journey of delicious discovery, leaving you excited for your next smoothie creation.

Crafting Your Champion Smoothie:

- Embrace the power of greens: Leafy greens like spinach, kale, or collard greens pack a nutrient punch without overpowering the flavor. Start with a handful of greens as your base to boost your smoothie's nutritional profile.

- Fruit Fiesta: Choose a variety of colorful fruits for sweetness and additional vitamins. Berries, bananas, mangoes, pineapples – the possibilities are endless! Combine different fruits to create unique flavor profiles and keep things interesting.

- Protein Powerhouse: Add a scoop of protein powder, Greek yogurt, or nut butter to your smoothie for sustained energy and muscle support. Experiment with different protein sources to find one that suits your taste and dietary needs.

- Healthy Fat Infusion: Don't shy away from healthy fats like avocado, chia seeds, or flaxseeds. They add creaminess, satiety, and essential nutrients to your smoothie, keeping you feeling satisfied and energized throughout the morning.

- Spice Up Your Life: Get creative with spices and herbs like ginger, cinnamon, turmeric, or mint. These add complexity to the flavor, boost your metabolism, and offer additional health benefits.

- Hydration Hero: Use water, unsweetened plant-based milk, or coconut water as your liquid base. Avoid sugary juices or sodas, as they will spike your blood sugar and leave you feeling tired later.

Remember, power-packed smoothies are not just about ingredients; they're about a mindset. Embrace the fun, the experimentation, and the joy of discovery. Turn your kitchen into a smoothie laboratory, your blender into a magical tool, and each morning into a celebration of deliciousness and well-being. So, grab your blender, unleash your inner culinary artist, and whip up a power-packed smoothie that fuels your body, ignites your energy, and sets the stage for a day of vibrant health and accomplishment. Cheers to mornings bursting with flavor, nutrition, and the power to seize the day!

Overnight Oats: A Make-Ahead Option for Busy Mornings

Rise and Shine, Not Scramble and Sigh: Overnight Oats – Your Make-Ahead Champion for Busy Mornings

Forget the frantic mornings and pre-dawn kitchen chaos. Your path to a calm, nourished start over 60 takes a delicious, well-planned turn with the overnight oats revolution. Imagine, not battling cereal boxes and burnt toast, but waking up to a prepped, protein-rich breakfast waiting patiently in your fridge. Picture, not sacrificing health for convenience, but relishing a cold, creamy concoction bursting with flavor and nutrition, setting the stage for a day of focus and well-being. Welcome to the world where overnight oats become your make-ahead champions, your fridge a culinary treasure trove, and every spoonful a celebration of morning ease and vibrant health.

Why do overnight oats hold the key to unlocking a tranquil, well-fueled start to your day? Here's the oat-tastic breakdown:

- Convenience Reigns Supreme: Ditch the rushed mornings and frantic breakfast routines. Overnight oats are the ultimate make-ahead breakfast solution. Simply mix your ingredients the night before, pop them in the fridge, and wake up to a ready-to-eat masterpiece. No cooking, no dishes, just a delicious, wholesome breakfast waiting to greet you.

- Nutritional Powerhouse in a Jar: Don't underestimate the humble oat. Overnight oats offer a protein-rich, fiber-packed base that keeps you feeling full and energized throughout the morning. Add nuts, seeds, fruits, and spices for a vitamin and mineral bonanza, transforming your breakfast into a nutritional powerhouse.

- Digestive Delight: Forget the heavy, greasy breakfasts that leave you feeling sluggish. Overnight oats are gentle on your digestive system, providing easily absorbed nutrients and fiber to keep things moving smoothly and comfortably all morning long.

- Time-Saving Superhero: Overnight oats are your busy morning's best friend. They save you precious time on those hectic days, allowing you to sleep in a little longer, enjoy a quiet read, or tackle your morning routine with newfound peace. No more frantic scrambling in the kitchen – your breakfast is ready the moment you are.

- Flavor and Customization Galore: Ditch the bland breakfasts and monotonous routines. Overnight oats offer a canvas for your culinary creativity. Experiment with different fruits, nuts, spices, and toppings – the possibilities are endless! Discover new flavor combinations, personalize your oatmeal to your unique preferences, and turn breakfast into a delightful culinary adventure.

Crafting Your Overnight Oats Masterpiece:

- Start with the oat-titude: Choose rolled oats for their perfect texture and overnight soaking capabilities. Experiment with quick oats for a smoother result or steel-cut oats for a chewier experience.

- Milk Matters: Use your favorite milk as the base – dairy, plant-based, or even nut milk! Each offers a unique flavor and nutritional profile, so choose the one that suits your taste and dietary needs.

- Protein Powerhouse: Add a scoop of protein powder, Greek yogurt, or nut butter for an extra energy boost and muscle support. Choose a protein source that complements the flavors of your chosen ingredients.

- Fruit Fiesta: Embrace the power of berries, bananas, mangoes, or any other fruit your heart desires. They add sweetness, vitamins, and a vibrant splash of color, making your breakfast even more appealing.

- Spice Up Your Life: Elevate your oatmeal with spices like cinnamon, nutmeg, ginger, or cardamom. These add complexity to the flavor, boost your metabolism, and offer additional health benefits.

- Go Nuts for Toppings: Don't forget the toppings! Sprinkle your oatmeal with nuts, seeds, granola, or even a drizzle of honey for added texture, flavor, and healthy fats.

Remember, overnight oats are not just about ingredients; they're about a mindset. Embrace the convenience, the customization, and the joy of waking up to a ready-made breakfast masterpiece. Turn your fridge into a culinary haven, your night owl hours into meal prep superpowers, and each morning into a celebration of calm, well-nourished mornings. So, stock up on your favorite oats, unleash your inner breakfast artist, and craft a jar of overnight oats that fuels your body, soothes your soul, and sets the stage for a day of productivity and well-being. Rise and shine, not scramble and sigh –

let overnight oats be your champion for a tranquil, delicious start to any day!

Scrambled Eggs with Spinach and Tomatoes: Protein, Vitamins, and Flavor

Rise and Shine with Sunshine on Your Plate: Scrambled Eggs with Spinach and Tomatoes – A Protein-Packed Feast for Champions

Forget the bland omelets and boring toast mornings. Your path to a vibrant, energized start over 60 takes a protein-rich, sun-kissed turn with the scrambled eggs with spinach and tomatoes symphony. Imagine, not battling rubbery yolks and greasy bacon, but savoring a fluffy, flavorful masterpiece bursting with vitamin-rich greens and juicy tomatoes. Picture, not settling for quick fixes and sugary cereals, but indulging in a protein powerhouse that fuels your body and ignites your senses, setting the stage for a day of well-being and accomplishment. Welcome to the world where scrambled eggs become your morning champions, your pan a culinary canvas, and every bite a celebration of deliciousness and vibrant health.

Why do scrambled eggs with spinach and tomatoes hold the key to unlocking a winning start to your day? Here's the protein-packed breakdown:

- Muscle-Building Champion: Eggs are nature's protein treasure trove, providing essential amino acids to build and maintain muscle mass, crucial for strength, mobility, and independence as we age. Each fluffy bite fuels your day with sustained energy, keeping you feeling strong and ready to tackle anything.

- Green Powerhouse: Spinach packs a nutrient punch, overflowing with vitamins A, C, and K, iron, and folate. This leafy green warrior boosts your immune system, supports bone health, and adds a delightful earthy touch to your scrambled eggs.

- Vitamin Explosion: Tomatoes are bursting with vitamins C, K, and lycopene, a powerful antioxidant that protects your cells from damage. Their vibrant color and juicy sweetness not only brighten your plate but also contribute to overall well-being.

- Flavor and Texture Symphony: This dish is a feast for both the eyes and the palate. The creamy richness of the eggs combines perfectly with the vibrant sweetness of the tomatoes and the subtle earthiness of the spinach, creating a flavor explosion that awakens your taste buds and sets the tone for a delightful day.

- Quick and Easy Preparation: Don't underestimate the simplicity of this dish. It takes just minutes to whip up, making it perfect for busy mornings or lazy weekends. With minimal ingredients and effortless cooking, you can enjoy a gourmet-worthy breakfast without breaking a sweat.

Crafting Your Scrambled Egg Masterpiece:

- Crack open the sunshine: Choose fresh, free-range eggs for optimal flavor and nutrition. Whisk them gently, incorporating air for a light and fluffy texture.

- Sauté the green goodness: Wilt your spinach in a pan with a drizzle of olive oil. This enhances its flavor and releases its beneficial nutrients.

- Embrace the sun-kissed sweetness: Dice your tomatoes and add them to the pan, letting them release their juices and mingle with the spinach.

- Gentle heat, fluffy magic: Pour your whisked eggs into the pan and let them cook slowly, stirring gently to create soft, creamy curds. Season with salt and pepper to taste.

- A touch of finesse: Plate your scrambled eggs, top them with a sprinkle of fresh herbs or a grated cheese, and let the vibrant colors and delicious aromas tempt your taste buds.

Remember, scrambled eggs with spinach and tomatoes are not just about ingredients; they're about an experience. Savor the process of cooking, appreciate the vibrant colors on your plate, and enjoy the burst of flavor in every bite. Turn your kitchen into a culinary sanctuary, your stovetop into an artist's palette, and each breakfast into a celebration of taste, well-being, and the simple joys of a nourishing start to the day. So, crack open some eggs, unleash your inner culinary artist, and whip up a plate of scrambled eggs with spinach and tomatoes that fuels your body, ignites your senses, and sets the stage for a day of sunshine on your plate and in your soul. Happy breakfasting!

Whole-Wheat Pancakes with Berries and Greek Yogurt: Sweet and Satisfying

Sweet Beginnings, Wholesome Choices: Unleashing the Power of Whole-Wheat Pancakes with Berries and Greek Yogurt

Forget the sugary cereal and calorie-laden pastries. Your path to a delicious, well-balanced start over 60 takes a warm, fluffy turn with the whole-wheat pancake symphony. Imagine, not battling syrup-soaked carbs and greasy bacon, but savoring a stack of golden brown delights bursting with the sweetness of berries and the creamy goodness of Greek yogurt. Picture, not succumbing to sugary cravings or empty calories, but indulging in a fiber-rich feast that satisfies your taste buds and nourishes your body, setting the stage for a day of vibrant energy and well-being. Welcome to the world where whole-wheat pancakes become your morning champions, your griddle a culinary canvas, and every bite a celebration of taste, texture, and vibrant health.

Why do whole-wheat pancakes with berries and Greek yogurt hold the key to unlocking a winning start to your day? Here's the sweet and satisfying breakdown:

- Fiber Powerhouse: Ditch the refined breakfast options and embrace the power of whole wheat. Packed with fiber, these pancakes keep you feeling full and satisfied throughout the morning, preventing unwanted cravings and promoting gut health. No mid-morning energy crashes – just sustained fuel to keep you going strong.

- Vitamin Explosion: Berries bring a vibrant splash of color and a potent dose of vitamins. From the antioxidant richness of blueberries to the vitamin C boost of strawberries, these tiny powerhouses add natural sweetness and protect your cells from damage. Each bite is a celebration of flavor and well-being.

- Protein Prowess: Greek yogurt is a champion of protein and healthy fats. This creamy companion adds a delightful tang to your pancakes, provides essential amino acids for muscle repair and maintenance, and keeps you feeling energized throughout the morning. No more breakfast fatigue – just steady fuel for your mind and body.

- Flavor and Texture Symphony: This dish is a delightful dance of textures and flavors. The fluffy pancakes contrast beautifully with the creamy yogurt and the juicy burst of berries. Each bite is a celebration of sweetness, tang, and a hint of nuttiness, leaving you wanting more.

- Versatile and Creative: Whole-wheat pancakes offer a blank canvas for culinary exploration. Experiment with different spices like cinnamon or nutmeg, add a drizzle of honey, or personalize your stack with different berries and toppings. Every breakfast becomes a joyful adventure in taste and creativity.

Crafting Your Whole-Wheat Pancake Masterpiece:

- Embrace the whole truth: Choose whole-wheat flour or a whole-wheat pancake mix for a fiber-rich base. You can even add a handful of oats for extra texture and nutritional punch.

- Wet wonderland: Whisk together milk, eggs, a touch of oil, and your favorite non-dairy milk or water. You can also add a banana for sweetness and additional moisture.

- Spiced up sensation: Don't forget the spices! Cinnamon, nutmeg, or even a hint of ginger add warmth and complexity to your pancake batter.

- Griddle goodness: Heat your griddle or pan over medium heat and lightly coat it with oil. Pour batter in small circles and let them cook until golden brown and bubbly.

- Berrylicious bliss: Pile your pancakes high, dollop on some Greek yogurt, and top it all off with a vibrant medley of fresh berries. A drizzle of honey or maple syrup is optional, as the natural sweetness of the berries often does the trick.

Remember, whole-wheat pancakes with berries and Greek yogurt are not just about ingredients; they're about an experience. Savor the process of battering, flipping, and stacking, appreciate the aroma that fills your kitchen, and enjoy the warm embrace of this wholesome breakfast in every bite. Turn your kitchen into a culinary haven, your griddle into an artist's palette, and each breakfast into a celebration of taste, well-being, and the simple joys of a satisfying start to the day. So, whip up a stack of whole-wheat pancakes, unleash your inner culinary artist, and savor a breakfast that fuels your body, delights your senses, and sets the stage for a day of vibrant health and contentment. Happy pancake-ing!

Chapter 8: Lunchtime Delights: Quick and Healthy Meals to Keep You Going

Salads with Colorful Vegetables and Lean Protein

Salad Symphonies: Unleashing the Power of Colorful Vegetables and Lean Protein for Vibrant Lunchtime Delights

Forget the wilted lettuce and greasy sandwiches. Your path to a delicious, well-fueled afternoon over 60 takes a vibrant, vitamin-packed turn with the transformative power of salads with colorful vegetables and lean protein. Imagine, not battling heavy midday meals and afternoon slumps, but savoring a symphony of textures and flavors bursting with the goodness of fresh vegetables and the satiating power of lean protein. Picture, not succumbing to unhealthy cravings or processed lunch options, but nourishing your body with a rainbow of colorful nutrients, setting the stage for an energized and productive afternoon. Welcome to the world where salads become your lunchtime champions, your plate a culinary canvas, and every bite a celebration of taste, health, and vibrant well-being.

Why do salads with colorful vegetables and lean protein hold the key to unlocking a winning lunchtime experience? Here's the symphony-in-a-salad breakdown:

- Vitamin and Mineral Explosion: Ditch the dull greens and embrace the rainbow. Load your salad with a variety of colorful vegetables like bell peppers, carrots, broccoli, leafy greens, tomatoes, and onions. Each hue represents a unique blend of vitamins, minerals, and antioxidants, fueling your body with a natural pharmacy of well-being.

- Fiber Powerhouse: Vegetables are champions of fiber, keeping you feeling full and satisfied throughout the afternoon. No more unhealthy snacking or mid-afternoon crashes – just sustained energy to power through your day.

- Lean Protein Prowess: Don't underestimate the power of protein. Add grilled chicken, salmon, tofu, or lentils to your salad for muscle support, satiety, and sustained energy. Choose lean protein sources to keep your meal healthy and balanced.

- Flavor and Texture Symphony: Salads are far from boring. Experiment with different combinations of vegetables, fruits, nuts, seeds, and cheeses to create unique flavor profiles and textural contrasts. Each bite becomes a delightful discovery, keeping your lunchtime routine exciting and enjoyable.

- Customization Craze: The beauty of salads is their versatility. Tailor your salad to your specific dietary needs and preferences. Gluten-free, vegan, dairy-free – the possibilities are endless! Embrace your individuality and create a salad that speaks to your taste buds and nutritional requirements.

Crafting Your Salad Masterpiece:

- Build your base: Start with a bed of mixed greens or your favorite leafy vegetables. Baby spinach, arugula, or even kale offer a delightful variety of textures and flavors.

- Rainbow Revolution: Choose at least 3-4 different colored vegetables to add an explosion of vitamins and minerals to your plate. Bell peppers, carrots, cucumbers, and tomatoes are perfect options for vibrant color and refreshing crunch.

- Protein Prowess: Don't skip the protein! Grill some chicken or salmon, bake tofu cubes, or sprinkle on lentils or chickpeas for sustained energy and muscle support.

- Flavor Fireworks: Enhance your salad with fruits like berries, oranges, or apples for sweetness and additional vitamins. Nuts, seeds, and cheeses add textural contrast and healthy fats, rounding out your meal with additional nutrients.

- Dressing Delight: Choose a light and flavorful dressing to tie everything together. Avoid sugary options and opt for vinaigrettes with fresh herbs or a simple lemon-olive oil combination.

Remember, salads with colorful vegetables and lean protein are not just about ingredients; they're about an experience. Transform your lunchtime into a celebration of vibrant colors, textures, and deliciousness. Make your kitchen a culinary studio, your bowl a blank canvas, and each bite a testament to your creative spirit and commitment to well-being. So, embrace the salad symphony, unleash your inner culinary artist, and create a lunchtime masterpiece that fuels your body, ignites your senses, and sets the stage for an energized and productive afternoon. Happy salad-ing!

Soups and Stews: Warm and Comforting, Packed with Goodness

Simmering Soulmates: Embracing the Warmth and Goodness of Soups and Stews for Comforting Lunchtime Delights

Forget the lukewarm leftovers and rushed sandwiches. Your path to a well-nourished, cozy afternoon over 60 takes a soul-warming turn with the enchanting power of soups and stews. Imagine, not battling bland lunches and afternoon chills, but savoring a steaming bowl of goodness filled with vibrant vegetables, tender meats, and the rich aroma of homemade love. Picture, not succumbing to unhealthy cravings or processed meals, but nourishing your body with a simmered symphony of flavors and nutrients, setting the stage for a contented and cozy afternoon. Welcome to the world where soups and stews become your lunchtime champions, your crockpot a culinary haven, and every spoonful a celebration of warmth, comfort, and vibrant well-being.

Why do soups and stews hold the key to unlocking a winning lunchtime experience? Here's the simmer-licious breakdown:

- Warmth on a Cool Day: Ditch the chills and embrace the comfort. Soups and stews offer a comforting hug on a cold day, warming your body from the inside out and soothing your soul with the gentle heat. No more afternoon shivers – just a cozy haven in every steaming bowl.

- Nutrient-Rich Symphony: Don't underestimate the power of a simmer. Stews and soups are treasure troves of vitamins, minerals, and antioxidants from vegetables, legumes, and lean proteins. Each spoonful nourishes your body with a natural pharmacy of well-being, keeping you healthy and energized.

- Fiber Powerhouse: Forget the heavy midday meals and afternoon slumps. The fiber-rich bounty of vegetables and legumes in soups and stews keeps you feeling full and satisfied throughout the afternoon. No more unhealthy snacking or mid-afternoon crashes – just sustained energy to power through your day.

- Digestive Delight: Ditch the greasy lunches and embrace the gentle touch. Soups and stews are easy on your digestive system, providing easily absorbed nutrients and soothing warmth that aids in digestion. No more post-lunch discomfort – just a gentle symphony of well-being in your belly.

- Flavor and Comfort Symphony: Soups and stews are culinary canvases for your creativity. Experiment with different spices, herbs, vegetables, and proteins to create unique flavor profiles and textures. Each new recipe becomes a journey of discovery, keeping your lunchtime routine exciting and comforting.

Crafting Your Simmering Masterpiece:

- Choose your adventure: Do you crave a creamy tomato bisque, a hearty lentil stew, or a vibrant vegetable minestrone? The possibilities are endless! Pick a recipe that suits your taste buds and dietary needs.

- Prep with joy: Spend some quality time chopping vegetables and browning meats beforehand. This prepares the stage for a quick and satisfying lunchtime feast.

- Simmer with love: Let your broth bubble away, infusing it with the flavors of herbs, spices, and vegetables. This slow, gentle process unlocks the magic of a homemade soup or stew.

- Embrace the leftovers: Soups and stews are champions of leftovers. Make a big batch on the weekend and enjoy satisfying lunches throughout the week. No more last-minute scrambling – just delicious, healthy comfort ready at your fingertips.

- Presentation matters: Don't underestimate the power of a beautiful bowl. Transfer your soup or stew to a vibrant bowl, garnish it with fresh herbs or a drizzle of olive oil, and let the presentation add to the cozy lunchtime experience.

Remember, soups and stews are not just about ingredients; they're about an experience. Transform your lunchtime into a celebration of warmth, comfort, and deliciousness. Make your kitchen a culinary haven, your crockpot a simmering storyteller, and each spoonful a testament to your love for home-cooked goodness and vibrant well-being. So, embrace the soup and stew symphony, unleash your inner culinary storyteller, and create a lunchtime masterpiece that warms your body, soothes your soul, and sets the stage for a contented and cozy afternoon. Happy simmering!

Turkey or Salmon Sandwiches on Whole-Grain Bread with Avocado

Sandwich Symphony: Unleashing the Power of Turkey or Salmon, Whole-Grain Bread, and Avocado for Flavorful, Nutritious Lunchtime Delights

Forget the soggy white bread and mystery lunch meat. Your path to a delicious, well-fueled afternoon over 60 takes a flavorful, textural turn with the sandwich symphony. Imagine, not battling cardboard crusts and greasy fillings, but savoring a delightful medley of flavors and textures bursting with the goodness of lean protein, whole-grain goodness, and creamy avocado. Picture, not succumbing to unhealthy cravings or processed lunch options, but nourishing your body with a balanced combination of protein, fiber, and healthy fats, setting the stage for an energized and productive afternoon. Welcome to the world where sandwiches become your lunchtime champions, your kitchen a culinary studio, and every bite a celebration of taste, health, and vibrant well-being.

Why do turkey or salmon sandwiches on whole-grain bread with avocado hold the key to unlocking a winning lunchtime experience? Here's the harmonious breakdown:

- Lean Protein Powerhouse: Ditch the fatty meats and embrace the champions of protein. Choose lean turkey slices or grilled salmon for sustained energy, muscle support, and satiety. No more afternoon hunger pangs – just sustained fuel to power through your day.

- Fiber Fiesta: Forget the white bread blues and embrace the whole-grain revolution. Opt for hearty whole-wheat, sprouted grain, or rye bread for a fiber-rich base that keeps you feeling full and satisfied throughout the afternoon. No more unhealthy snacking or mid-afternoon crashes – just sustained energy without the bloat.

- Healthy Fat Harmony: Don't shy away from healthy fats. Spread creamy avocado on your bread for a delicious source of monounsaturated fats, promoting satiety, heart health, and skin-glowing goodness. Each bite becomes a delightful dance of creamy avocado against the protein and fiber, keeping your taste buds singing and your well-being soaring.

- Flavor and Texture Symphony: Sandwiches are far from boring. Experiment with different toppings like crunchy lettuce, juicy tomatoes, pickled onions, or fresh herbs to create unique flavor profiles and textural contrasts. Each new creation becomes a culinary adventure, keeping your lunchtime routine exciting and delicious.

- Customization Craze: The beauty of sandwiches is their versatility. Tailor your meal to your specific dietary needs and preferences. Gluten-free, low-carb, vegetarian – the possibilities are endless! Embrace your individuality and create a sandwich that speaks to your taste buds and nutritional requirements.

Crafting Your Sandwich Masterpiece:

- Choose your protein champion: Do you crave the classic taste of roast turkey or the rich omega-3 goodness of grilled salmon? Pick a protein that suits your taste and nutritional needs.

- Bread bonanza: Explore the world of whole-grain breads. Consider different textures and flavors, like sprouted grain for nuttiness or rye for a tangy twist. Find a bread that makes your taste buds sing!

- Avocado adoration: Choose a perfectly ripe avocado for creamy perfection. Mash it slightly or slice it thin, depending on your preference. Let the smooth richness of avocado elevate your sandwich to new heights.

- Topping tango: Don't underestimate the power of toppings! Add crunchy lettuce, juicy tomatoes, pickled onions, or fresh herbs for textural and flavor contrasts. Let each bite be a delightful explosion of sensations.

- Presentation matters: Ditch the plastic wrap and embrace the beautiful bowl. Transfer your sandwich to a vibrant plate, add a side of colorful salad or fruit, and let the presentation add to the joyful lunchtime experience.

Remember, turkey or salmon sandwiches on whole-grain bread with avocado are not just about ingredients; they're about an experience. Transform your lunchtime into a celebration of flavorful combinations, textural delights, and vibrant health. Make your kitchen a culinary studio, your knife a brush, and each bite a testament to your creative spirit and commitment to well-being. So, embrace the sandwich symphony, unleash your inner culinary artist, and create a lunchtime masterpiece that fuels your body, ignites your senses, and sets the stage for an energized and productive afternoon. Happy sandwich-ing!

Lentil Bowls with Roasted Vegetables and Herbs

From Humble Lentil to Vibrant Feast: Unleashing the Power of Lentil Bowls with Roasted Vegetables and Herbs for Delicious and Nutritious Lunchtime Delights

Forget the same old salad or microwaved leftovers. Your path to a flavorful, well-fueled afternoon over 60 takes a deliciously global turn with the transformative power of lentil bowls. Imagine, not battling bland plates and afternoon slumps, but savoring a vibrant fiesta of textures and flavors bursting with the protein-packed goodness of lentils and the sun-kissed sweetness of roasted vegetables. Picture, not succumbing to unhealthy cravings or processed meals, but nourishing your body with a symphony of vitamins, minerals, and fiber, setting the stage for an energized and productive afternoon. Welcome to the world where lentil bowls become your lunchtime champions, your oven a culinary canvas, and every bite a celebration of deliciousness, diversity, and vibrant well-being.

Why do lentil bowls with roasted vegetables and herbs hold the key to unlocking a winning lunchtime experience? Here's the bowl-ilicious breakdown:

- Protein Powerhouse: Ditch the animal protein and embrace the champions of the plant world. Lentils are nature's protein treasure trove, packing each bite with essential amino acids for muscle repair and maintenance. No more afternoon fatigue – just sustained energy to keep you going strong.

- Fiber Fiesta: Forget the empty carbs and embrace the gut-friendly goodness. Lentils are bursting with fiber, keeping you feeling full and satisfied throughout the afternoon. No more unhealthy snacking or mid-afternoon crashes – just sustained satiety and happy digestion.

- Vitamin and Mineral Explosion: Dive into a rainbow of roasted vegetables! Bell peppers, carrots, broccoli, onions, and sweet potatoes offer a potent dose of vitamins, minerals, and antioxidants, fueling your body with a natural pharmacy of well-being. Each bite becomes a celebration of health and vibrant hues.

- Flavor and Texture Symphony: Lentil bowls are far from boring. Experiment with different spices and herbs like cumin, coriander, turmeric, and fresh parsley to create unique flavor profiles and build layers of complexity. Each new recipe becomes a culinary adventure, keeping your lunchtime routine exciting and delicious.

- Endless Customization Craze: The beauty of lentil bowls is their versatility. Tailor your meal to your specific dietary needs and preferences. Vegan, gluten-free, Mediterranean-inspired – the possibilities are endless! Embrace your individuality and create a bowl that speaks to your taste buds and nutritional requirements.

Crafting Your Lentil Bowl Masterpiece:

- Lentil love: Choose your favorite lentil variety! Brown lentils offer a hearty texture, while green lentils bring a delicate earthiness. Cook them according to your preferred method, letting them simmer in flavorful broth for extra oomph.

- Vegetable fiesta: Roast your chosen vegetables until tender and caramelized. Play with different colors, textures, and flavors to create a vibrant medley. Bell peppers and onions add sweetness, broccoli brings a touch of earthiness, and sweet potatoes offer a creamy twist.

- Spiced-up sensation: Don't forget the spices! Experiment with different combinations to create your signature blend. Cumin, coriander, turmeric, and cayenne pepper offer warmth and depth of flavor, while fresh parsley adds a vibrant parsley kick.

- Herb haven: Don't underestimate the power of fresh herbs. Sprinkle your bowl with chopped parsley, cilantro, or dill for an extra layer of flavor and a pop of freshness.

- Topping tango: Get creative with toppings! Drizzle with olive oil, sprinkle with toasted nuts or seeds, add a dollop of tahini or Greek yogurt, or even crumble some feta cheese for a tangy twist. Let each bite be a delightful discovery.

Remember, lentil bowls with roasted vegetables and herbs are not just about ingredients; they're about an experience. Transform your lunchtime into a celebration of global flavors, textures, and vibrant health. Make your kitchen a culinary studio, your oven a magical transformation chamber, and each bite a testament to your creative spirit and commitment to well-being. So, embrace the lentil bowl symphony, unleash your inner culinary artist, and create a lunchtime masterpiece that fuels your body, ignites your senses, and sets the stage for an energized and productive afternoon. Happy bowl eating!

Chapter 9: Dinnertime Feasts: Delicious and Nourishing Meals for Family and Friends

One-Pan Wonders: Easy Clean-Up, Delicious Results

Ditch the Dishwashing Drama: Unleashing the Power of One-Pan Wonders for Delicious and Nourishing Dinnertime Feasts with Family and Friends

Forget the post-dinner dishwashing vortex and the frantic pre-meal prep rush. Your path to a stress-free, flavorful evening over 60 takes a magically efficient turn with the transformative power of one-pan wonders. Imagine, not battling mountains of dirty dishes and recipe chaos, but savoring a beautifully balanced feast bursting with flavors and aromas, all nestled on a single pan. Picture, not sacrificing family time or evening relaxation for culinary struggles, but enjoying a seamless transition from kitchen to table, filled with laughter, conversation, and the simple joy of sharing a well-cooked meal. Welcome to the world where one-pan wonders become your dinnertime champions, your oven a culinary sanctuary, and every bite a celebration of deliciousness, togetherness, and effortless well-being.

Why do one-pan wonders hold the key to unlocking a winning dinnertime experience? Here's the dish-washing-defying breakdown:

- Minimal Mess, Maximum Flavor: Ditch the pots and pans pandemonium and embrace the magic of one-pan simplicity. Fewer tools translate to less cleaning, freeing up your precious time for what truly matters – enjoying your meal and connecting with loved ones. No more scrubbing and soaking – just a single pan to wash and a peaceful post-dinner glow.

- Effortless Efficiency, Delicious Results: Don't underestimate the power of simplicity. One-pan meals often require minimal prep and cooking time, making them perfect for busy weeknights or casual gatherings. Toss together your ingredients, let the oven work its magic, and emerge with a dish that's bursting with flavor and perfectly cooked. No more hours in the kitchen – just effortless culinary triumphs and more time for laughter and conversation.

- Variety and Versatility: One-pan doesn't equal boring! The possibilities are endless, from vibrant sheet pan roasted vegetables and tender protein combinations to bubbling casseroles and one-pot pastas. Explore ethnic cuisines, experiment with seasonal ingredients, and create dishes that tantalize your taste buds and inspire culinary adventures. Each night becomes a delicious journey, keeping your dinner routine exciting and full of surprises.

- Stress-Free Sharing, Joyful Gathering: Ditch the pre-meal frenzy and embrace the relaxed social ease of one-pan wonders. These meals are designed for sharing, encouraging conversation and laughter around the table. No more hovering in the kitchen while guests wait – just a simple, beautiful dish that invites everyone to gather, connect, and celebrate the joy of a home-cooked meal.

- Healthy and Holistic: One-pan doesn't have to mean greasy or unhealthy. Opt for lean protein choices, vibrant vegetables, and whole grains to create well-balanced dishes that nourish your body and satisfy your soul. Let each meal be a celebration of flavor and well-being, leaving you feeling energized and content.

Crafting Your One-Pan Masterpiece:

- Choose your adventure: Do you crave a Mediterranean-inspired sheet pan feast of roasted chicken, vegetables, and olives? Or are you dreaming of a comforting one-pot sausage and lentil stew? Pick a recipe that suits your taste buds and dietary needs.

- Prep with joy: Spend some quality time chopping vegetables, trimming proteins, and mixing sauces beforehand. This simple prep sets the stage for a seamless transition from oven to table.

- Let the oven be your hero: Trust the magic of your oven. Toss your ingredients together, drizzle with oil and spices, and let the heat work its magic. No need for constant hovering – just check occasionally and bask in the delicious aromas filling your kitchen.

- Presentation matters: Don't underestimate the power of a beautiful plate. Transfer your one-pan creation to a serving dish, garnish with fresh herbs or a squeeze of lemon, and let the presentation add to the joyful dinnertime experience.

- Embrace the leftovers: One-pan wonders excel at leftovers! Enjoy your meal tonight, then store the rest for a quick and delicious lunch the next day. No more last-minute scrambling – just healthy, flavorful leftovers ready at your fingertips.

Remember, one-pan wonders are not just about ingredients; they're about an experience. Transform your dinnertime into a celebration of flavor, efficiency, and shared joy. Make your kitchen a culinary haven, your oven a magical storyteller, and each bite a testament to your love for simple pleasures and vibrant well-being. So, embrace the one-pan symphony, unleash your inner culinary storyteller, and create a dinnertime masterpiece that brings your family and friends together, nourishes your bodies, and warms your hearts. Happy one-panning!

Sheet Pan Dinners: Roast Chicken with Vegetables, Salmon with Herbs

Sheet Pan Symphony: Unleashing the Power of Roast Chicken and Salmon with Vegetables for Effortless and Flavorful Dinnertime Feasts

Forget the pre-dinner frenzy and post-dishwashing drama. Your path to a stress-free, flavorful evening over 60 takes a vibrant, oven-roasted turn with the transformative power of the sheet pan symphony. Imagine, not battling greasy splatters and mountains of dirty dishes, but savoring a beautifully balanced feast nestled on a single pan, bursting with the golden goodness of roast chicken or the succulent richness of salmon, all accompanied by a vibrant medley of caramelized vegetables. Picture, not sacrificing precious evening hours in the kitchen or forgoing family time for culinary struggles, but enjoying a seamless transition from kitchen to table, filled with laughter, conversation, and the simple joy of sharing a well-cooked meal. Welcome to the world where sheet pan dinners become your dinnertime champions, your oven a culinary sanctuary, and every bite a celebration of deliciousness, togetherness, and effortless well-being.

Why do sheet pan dinners with roast chicken or salmon and vegetables hold the key to unlocking a winning dinnertime experience? Here's the harmony on a single pan breakdown:

- Minimal Mess, Maximum Flavor: Ditch the pots and pans pandemonium and embrace the magic of one-pan simplicity. Fewer tools translate to less cleaning, freeing up your precious time for what truly matters – enjoying your meal and connecting with loved ones. No more scrubbing and soaking – just a single pan to wash and a peaceful post-dinner glow.

- Effortless Efficiency, Delicious Results: Don't underestimate the power of simplicity. Sheet pan dinners often require minimal prep and cooking time, making them perfect for busy weeknights or casual gatherings. Toss together your ingredients, let the oven work its magic, and emerge with a dish that's bursting with flavor and perfectly cooked. No more hours in the kitchen – just effortless culinary triumphs and more time for laughter and conversation.

- Variety and Versatility: One pan doesn't equal boring! The possibilities are endless, from Mediterranean-inspired chicken with vibrant peppers and onions to Asian-style salmon with ginger and bok choy. Explore global flavors, experiment with seasonal vegetables, and create dishes that tantalize your taste buds and inspire culinary adventures. Each night becomes a delicious journey, keeping your dinner routine exciting and full of surprises.

- Stress-Free Sharing, Joyful Gathering: Ditch the pre-meal frenzy and embrace the relaxed social ease of sheet pan dinners. These meals are designed for sharing, encouraging conversation and laughter around the table. No more hovering in the kitchen while guests wait – just a simple, beautiful dish that invites everyone to gather, connect, and celebrate the joy of a home-cooked meal.

- Healthy and Holistic: Sheet pan doesn't have to mean greasy or unhealthy. Opt for lean protein choices, vibrant vegetables, and whole grains to create well-balanced dishes that nourish your body and satisfy your soul. Let each meal be a celebration of flavor and well-being, leaving you feeling energized and content.

Crafting Your Sheet Pan Masterpiece:

- Choose your champion: Do you crave the classic comfort of roast chicken with rosemary and potatoes, or are you dreaming of a lighter, citrusy salmon with fennel and asparagus? Pick a recipe that suits your taste buds and dietary needs.

- Prep with joy: Spend some quality time chopping vegetables, seasoning your protein, and mixing simple sauces beforehand. This simple prep sets the stage for a seamless transition from oven to table.

- Let the oven be your hero: Trust the magic of your oven. Arrange your ingredients on a single pan, drizzle with healthy oils and spices, and let the heat work its magic. No need for constant hovering – just check occasionally and bask in the delicious aromas filling your kitchen.

- Presentation matters: Don't underestimate the power of a beautiful plate. Transfer your sheet pan creation to a serving dish, garnish with fresh herbs or a squeeze of lemon, and let the presentation add to the joyful dinnertime experience.

- Embrace the leftovers: Sheet pan dinners excel at leftovers! Enjoy your meal tonight, then store the rest for a quick and delicious lunch the next day. No more last-minute scrambling – just healthy, flavorful leftovers ready at your fingertips.

Remember, sheet pan dinners are not just about ingredients; they're about an experience. Transform your dinnertime into a celebration of flavor, efficiency, and shared joy. Make your kitchen a culinary haven, your oven a magical storyteller, and each bite a testament to your love for simple pleasures and vibrant well-being. So, embrace the sheet pan symphony, unleash your inner culinary storyteller, and create a dinnertime masterpiece that brings your family and friends together, nourishes your bodies, and warms your hearts. Happy sheet-panning!

Bonus Tips:

- For extra crispy chicken skin, pat the chicken dry before seasoning and roasting.

- Play with textures: Mix and match your vegetables to create contrasting textures. Crispy roasted potatoes pair beautifully with tender asparagus, while sweet potato wedges add a creamy counterpoint to crunchy onions.

- Don't be afraid of spices: Experiment with different spice combinations to create unique flavor profiles. A touch of smoked paprika and cumin adds warmth to roast chicken, while a citrusy marinade with ginger and garlic elevates salmon to new heights.

- Go global: Take your taste buds on a journey! Experiment with Mediterranean herbs like oregano and thyme for roast chicken, or try a Moroccan-inspired salmon with preserved lemons and olives. The possibilities are endless!

- Get creative with toppings: A simple dollop of hummus adds a Mediterranean twist to roasted vegetables, while a drizzle of tahini or sriracha sauce can add a spicy kick. Fresh herbs like parsley or cilantro offer a bright finishing touch.

- Make it your own: The beauty of sheet pan dinners is their versatility. Don't be afraid to adjust ingredients and spices to suit your preferences and dietary needs. Whether you prefer vegetarian options or want to add your favorite grains, the possibilities are endless!

Beyond the Sheet Pan:

- Soup for the Soul: Don't let the leftovers go to waste! Roast your vegetables and protein the night before, then toss them into a pot with some broth and simmer for a quick and delicious soup the next day.

- Salad Remix: Leftover roasted vegetables add flavor and texture to a simple salad. Chop them up, toss them with greens, and drizzle with a vinaigrette for a light and refreshing lunch.

- Sandwich Sensation: Leftover chicken or salmon makes the perfect filling for a hearty sandwich. Add some avocado, lettuce, and your favorite condiments for a delicious and satisfying meal.

With a little creativity and these handy tips, sheet pan dinners can become your go-to for creating stress-free, flavorful meals that your whole family will love. So get ready to embrace the symphony of the sheet pan, unleash your inner culinary maestro, and create dinnertime memories that are as delicious as they are effortless. Happy cooking!

Slow Cooker Creations: Set and Forget, Enjoy Flavorful Meals

Savor the Simmer: Unveiling the Magic of Slow Cooker Creations for Effortless and Flavorful Dinnertime Feasts

Forget the pre-dinner frenzy and chaotic kitchen dance. Your path to a soul-warming, fuss-free evening over 60 takes a slow, aromatic turn with the transformative power of slow cooker creations. Imagine, not battling greasy splatters and frantic recipe juggling, but savoring a beautifully simmered feast bursting with tenderness and flavor, all crafted with minimal effort in your trusty ceramic crockpot. Picture, not sacrificing precious quality time with loved ones for culinary struggles, but settling back with a glass of wine as your slow cooker works its magic, filling your home with the promise of a delicious reward. Welcome to the world where slow cooker creations become your dinnertime champions, your kitchen a comforting haven, and every bite a celebration of slow-simmered goodness, shared laughter, and effortless well-being.

Why do slow cooker creations hold the key to unlocking a winning dinnertime experience? Here's the simmer-licious breakdown:

- Set and Forget, Savor the Joy: Ditch the constant kitchen hovering and embrace the magic of "set it and forget it." Toss your ingredients in the pot, add a touch of love, and let the gentle heat work its magic while you go about your day. No more stressing over stir-frying or flipping pancakes – just delicious anticipation and the joy of returning to a home filled with inviting aromas.

- Effortless Efficiency, Flavorful Triumphs: Don't underestimate the power of simplicity. Slow cooker meals often require minimal prep and active cooking time, making them perfect for busy weeknights or relaxed gatherings. No more chopping through mountains of vegetables – just throw in the essentials, let the slow cooker coax out the flavors, and emerge with a dish that's bursting with tenderness and depth.

- Variety and Versatility: One pot doesn't equal boring! The possibilities are endless, from rich and comforting beef stews and aromatic curries to tender pulled pork and melt-in-your-mouth chicken casseroles. Explore global cuisines, experiment with seasonal ingredients, and create dishes that tantalize your taste buds and inspire culinary adventures. Each night becomes a delicious journey, keeping your dinner routine exciting and full of surprises.

- Stress-Free Sharing, Warm Gatherings: Ditch the pre-meal frenzy and embrace the relaxed social ease of slow cooker feasts. These meals are designed for gathering and unwinding, encouraging conversation and laughter around the table. No more last-minute plating or pot juggling – just a simple, steaming pot inviting everyone to gather, connect, and celebrate the joy of a home-cooked meal.

- Healthy and Holistic: Slow cooking doesn't have to mean calorie-laden or greasy. Opt for lean protein choices, vibrant vegetables, and whole grains to create well-balanced dishes that nourish your body and satisfy your soul. Let each meal be a celebration of flavor and well-being, leaving you feeling energized and content.

Crafting Your Slow Cooker Masterpiece:

- Choose your culinary journey: Do you crave the hearty comfort of a classic beef stew, or are you dreaming of a Thai-inspired curry with coconut milk and vegetables? Pick a recipe that suits your taste buds and dietary needs.

- Prep with joy: Spend some quality time chopping vegetables, browning meats, and mixing simple sauces beforehand. This simple prep sets the stage for a seamless transition from pot to table.

- Let the simmer be your storyteller: Trust the gentle magic of your slow cooker. Layer your ingredients, add your aromatics, and let the low heat work its magic. No need for constant hovering – just check occasionally and bask in the anticipation of a delicious reward.

- Presentation matters: Don't underestimate the power of a beautiful plate. Transfer your slow cooker creation to a serving dish, garnish with fresh herbs or a dollop of yogurt, and let the presentation add to the joyful dinnertime experience.

- Embrace the leftovers: Slow cooker meals excel at leftovers! Enjoy your feast tonight, then store the rest for a quick and delicious lunch the next day. No more last-minute scrambling – just healthy, flavorful leftovers ready at your fingertips.

Remember, slow cooker creations are not just about ingredients; they're about an experience. Transform your dinnertime into a celebration of slow-simmered goodness, shared laughter, and effortless well-being. Make your kitchen a comforting haven, your slow cooker a culinary storyteller, and each bite a testament to your love for simple pleasures and vibrant living. So, embrace the slow cooker symphony, unleash your inner culinary artisan, and create a dinnertime masterpiece that warms your body, soothes your soul, and brings your loved ones together. Happy simmering!

Bonus Tips:

- Brown your meats for extra flavor. This step adds depth and richness to your dish, even though it's not always essential in a slow cooker.

- Play with layers and textures: Don't just dump everything in and walk away! Arrange your ingredients with intention, layering vegetables and meats for even cooking and contrasting textures. Crispy chickpeas can add bite to a slow-cooked stew, while tender root vegetables create a velvety contrast to lean protein.

- Don't be afraid of spices: Let your slow cooker become a flavor incubator! Experiment with different spice combinations to infuse your dishes with warmth, depth, and complexity. A touch of smoked paprika and cumin can transform a simple chicken stew, while a Moroccan-inspired tagine with cinnamon and ginger will transport your taste buds to exotic lands.

- Go global: Take your slow cooker on a culinary adventure! Explore the world through fragrant curries, robust stews, and comforting casseroles from different cultures. A slow cooker is your passport to delicious discoveries, all nestled within the cozy confines of your own kitchen.

- Get creative with toppings: A simple dollop of pesto can add a fresh twist to a slow-cooked lentil dish, while a dollop of Greek yogurt or tahini can turn a roasted vegetable medley into a Mediterranean masterpiece. Fresh herbs like parsley, cilantro, or dill offer a final touch of vibrant flavor and color.

- Make it your own: The beauty of slow cookers is their versatility. Don't be afraid to adjust ingredients and spices to suit your preferences and dietary needs. Whether you prefer vegetarian options or want to add your favorite grains, pulses, or even fruits, the possibilities are endless!

Beyond the Slow Cooker:

- Soup Sensation: Don't let the leftovers go to waste! Pulse your slow-cooked creation with some broth for a quick and healthy soup. Leftover pulled pork adds smoky depth to a black bean soup, while roasted vegetables transform into a creamy butternut squash bisque.

- Sandwich Surprise: Leftover slow-cooked meats are the perfect filling for a hearty sandwich. Shredded chicken goes beautifully with avocado and pesto on toasted ciabatta, while pulled pork shines in a Cuban-style sandwich with roasted onions and pickles.

- Salad Remix: Leftover slow-cooked vegetables add flavor and texture to a simple salad. Roast them before adding them to the pot, then chop them up and toss them with greens and your favorite dressing for a light and delicious lunch.

With a little creativity and these handy tips, slow cooker creations can become your go-to for creating stress-free, flavorful meals that your whole family will love. So get ready to embrace the simmer of the slow cooker, unleash your inner culinary alchemist, and create dinnertime memories that are as comforting as they are delicious. Happy slow cooking!

Let the gentle heat of your slow cooker be your muse, your kitchen your canvas, and your family and friends your joyful culinary companions. Bon appétit!

Vegetarian Chili: Hearty, Satisfying, and Nutrient-Rich

Beyond Beans and Corn: Unlocking the Symphony of Flavor in Vegetarian Chili for Hearty, Satisfying, and Nutrient-Rich Dinners

Forget the bland, bean-laden stereotype of vegetarian chili. Your path to a vibrant, soul-warming dinner over 60 takes a flavorful, plant-powered turn with the transformative magic of vegetarian chili. Imagine, not settling for a watery bowl of mush, but savoring a rich, complex symphony of textures and tastes, bursting with the goodness of roasted vegetables, tender legumes, and fragrant spices, all nestled in a simmering broth that warms your body and fuels your soul. Picture, not sacrificing deliciousness or satisfying fullness for a meat-free meal, but creating a dish that rivals any carnivore's wildest dreams, leaving smiles of contentment around the table and smiles of well-being on your face. Welcome to the world where vegetarian chili becomes your dinnertime champion, your kitchen a culinary playground, and every bite a celebration of vibrant vegetables, bold spices, and shared joy.

Why does vegetarian chili hold the key to unlocking a winning dinnertime experience? Here's the flavorful breakdown:

- Hearty Satisfaction, Not Bland Compromise: Ditch the notion that vegetarian means flimsy. This chili embraces hearty grains like quinoa or brown rice, protein-packed legumes like lentils and chickpeas, and the creamy richness of sweet potatoes or butternut squash, creating a dish that leaves you feeling comfortably full and deliciously satisfied.

No more post-dinner hunger pangs – just sustained energy and a happy body.

- Flavor Symphony, Not Monotony: One-dimensional is not in this chili's vocabulary. We're talking layers of caramelized onions and smoky bell peppers, earthy mushrooms and fragrant spices, a touch of acidity from tomatoes and a hint of sweetness from roasted vegetables, all simmered in a flavorful broth that evolves with every spoonful. Each bite becomes a culinary adventure, keeping your taste buds engaged and your cravings satiated.

- Nutrient Riches, Not Empty Calories: This chili is a plant-based powerhouse! Bursting with vitamins, minerals, fiber, and antioxidants from a rainbow of vegetables and legumes, it nourishes your body while tantalizing your taste buds. No more guilt-ridden indulgence – just healthy happiness in every bowl.

- Versatility and Customization: One pot doesn't equal boring! Vegetarian chili welcomes improvisation. Swap black beans for kidney beans, add a touch of chipotle spice for heat, or toss in your favorite seasonal vegetables for a unique twist. Each version becomes a personal expression, keeping your dinner routine exciting and full of creative possibilities.

- Warmth and Connection, Not Isolation in the Kitchen: This chili is meant for sharing. Simmer a big pot, gather your loved ones around the table, and invite laughter and conversation to flow as freely as the broth. No more rushed meals eaten on the go – just a comforting ritual of warmth, connection, and shared enjoyment.

Crafting Your Vegetarian Chili Masterpiece:

- Choose your texture symphony: Do you crave a chunky chili with distinct bites of beans and vegetables, or a smoother version with creamy sweet potato or butternut squash? Play with textures to create a mouthwatering contrast.

- Prepare with joy, not dread: Embrace the chopping and prepping as a mindful culinary ritual. Dice your vegetables, toast your spices, and simmer your broth with love. This sets the stage for a delicious journey from kitchen to table.

- Let the heat be your storyteller: Trust the magic of your simmering pot. Layer your ingredients, add your aromatics, and let the gentle heat work its magic. No need for constant hovering – just check occasionally and bask in the intoxicating aromas filling your kitchen.

- Presentation matters, even in a bowl: Don't underestimate the power of a beautiful serving. Transfer your chili to a colorful bowl, garnish with fresh cilantro or avocado slices, and let the presentation add to the joyful dinnertime experience.

- Embrace the leftovers, don't fear them: This chili is a champion of leftovers! Enjoy a big bowl tonight, then store the rest for a quick and delicious lunch the next day. No more last-minute scrambling – just healthy, flavorful leftovers ready at your fingertips.

Remember, vegetarian chili is not just about ingredients; it's about an experience. Transform your dinnertime into a celebration of vibrant flavors, textures, and shared well-being. Make your kitchen a culinary laboratory, your simmering pot a storyteller, and each bite a testament to your love for simple pleasures and mindful living. So, embrace the chili symphony, unleash your inner culinary artist, and create a dinnertime masterpiece that warms your body, ignites your senses, and brings your loved ones together. Happy chili-ing!

Bonus Tips:

- Roast your vegetables for extra depth of flavor: Roasting onions, peppers, and root vegetables before adding them to the chili unlocks a caramelized sweetness and rich smokiness that takes your dish

- Don't shy away from spice: Get creative with your spice blend! Go classic with smoked paprika and cumin, add a touch of warmth with chili powder and cayenne, or explore international flavors with garam masala or harissa. Remember, a little spice goes a long way!

- Play with protein sources: Expand your horizons beyond black beans! Lentils, chickpeas, quinoa, and even tempeh can all add unique textures and protein punches to your chili. Explore different combinations and find your favorites.

- Go global with flavor inspiration: Take your taste buds on a journey! Use Mexican chipotle peppers for a smoky kick, Moroccan ras el hanout for warm earthiness, or Indian curry powder for a vibrant twist. The world is your culinary oyster!

- Top it off for personalization: Let everyone personalize their chili experience! Offer a selection of toppings like chopped onions, grated cheese, fresh herbs, sour cream, avocado slices, or even tortilla chips for scooping.

- Make it your own: The beauty of vegetarian chili is its adaptability. Don't be afraid to adjust ingredients and spices to suit your tastes and dietary needs. Add chopped kale for an extra boost of greens, swap quinoa for brown rice, or even sneak in some grated zucchini for a hidden veggie surprise. The possibilities are endless!

Beyond the Pot:

- Chili Leftovers, Reborn: Don't let the leftovers languish! Leftover chili can be transformed into delicious quesadillas, stuffed into baked potatoes, or even whirled into a hearty soup with some additional broth. Think beyond the bowl and unleash your culinary creativity.

- Chili Night, Fiesta Edition: Turn your vegetarian chili into a full-blown fiesta! Serve it with warm tortillas, crunchy corn chips, a rainbow of chopped vegetables, and a selection of salsas and guacamole. Let the fun and flavor flow!

- Chili for the Soul: Don't forget the power of comfort food! This chili is perfect for cold winter nights, rainy afternoons, or any time you need a warm hug in a bowl. So cozy up, gather your loved ones, and let the chili nourish your body and soul.

With a little creativity and these handy tips, vegetarian chili can become your go-to for creating flavorful, nutritious, and satisfying meals that your whole family will love. So get ready to embrace the warmth of the simmering pot, unleash your inner culinary alchemist, and create dinnertime memories that are as vibrant and comforting as your chili itself. Happy cooking, happy sharing, and happy chili-ing!

Chapter 10: Healthy Snacks to Keep Hunger at Bay:

Fruits with Nut Butter: A Classic Combination for Satiety

Beyond Peanut Butter and Bananas: Unveiling the Symphony of Flavors and Nutrients in Fruits with Nut Butter for Delicious and Satiating Snacks

Forget the same old, same old. Ditch the stale bag of chips and the sugary cookies. Your path to a vibrant, taste-bud-tingling, and health-conscious snacking experience takes a refreshingly natural turn with the classic, yet endlessly inventive, combination of fruits with nut butter. Imagine, not settling for a monotonous nibble, but savoring a burst of juicy sweetness punctuated by creamy richness, all nestled in a symphony of textures and flavors that ignite your senses and nourish your body. Picture, not succumbing to hunger pangs or afternoon slumps, but enjoying a snack that keeps you feeling satisfied and energized, leaving you with a smile on your face and a glow of well-being radiating from within. Welcome to the world where fruits with nut butter become your snacktime champions, your kitchen a playground of possibilities, and every bite a celebration of nature's bounty, culinary creativity, and effortless well-being.

Why does this seemingly simple combination hold the key to unlocking a winning snack time experience? Here's the delicious breakdown:

- Satiety Symphony: Ditch the fleeting sugar highs and crash-and-burn energy dips. Fruits and nut butter are a match made in satiety heaven. The natural sugars in fruits provide a quick burst of energy, while the healthy fats and protein in nut butter offer sustained fullness, keeping you satisfied for longer and curbing those unwelcome hunger pangs. No more pre-dinner snack raids – just healthy energy and focus throughout the day.

- Flavor Fiesta: One combination does not equal boring! This dynamic duo welcomes endless exploration. Tart apples marry beautifully with the richness of almond butter, juicy berries dance with the nutty creaminess of cashew butter, and tropical mangoes tango with the subtle earthiness of peanut butter. Each pairing becomes a culinary adventure, keeping your taste buds engaged and your snack routine exciting.

- Nutrient Powerhouse: This snack packs a nutritional punch! Fruits burst with vitamins, minerals, and antioxidants, while nut butter offers a bounty of healthy fats, protein, and essential nutrients. No more empty calories or guilt-ridden indulgences – just a healthy snack that nourishes your body and fuels your well-being.

- Convenience and Versatility: This snack is your anytime, anywhere companion. No fancy equipment or complicated recipes needed! Grab a few slices of your favorite fruit, spread on some nut butter, and voila – a delicious and nourishing snack ready in seconds. Whether you're on the go, at work, or relaxing at home, this dynamic duo has your back (and your stomach) covered.

- Mindful and Joyful Experience: This snack is not just about fuel; it's about pleasure. Savor the juicy snap of the fruit, the creamy richness of the nut butter, the interplay of textures, and the symphony of flavors dancing on your tongue.

Embrace the mindful act of preparing and enjoying each bite, transforming your snack break into a mini-ritual of self-care and joy.

Crafting Your Personal Fruit and Nut Butter Masterpiece:

- Choose your flavor adventure: Do you crave the classic comfort of apple slices dipped in almond butter, or are you dreaming of a tropical escape with mango chunks and cashew butter? Explore different fruit and nut butter combinations, finding pairings that tantalize your taste buds and spark your culinary curiosity.

- Get creative with textures: Go beyond the expected! Slice your fruit into spears, cubes, or wedges, or even roast them for a warm and caramelized twist. Play with different nut butters: smooth, crunchy, or even flavored varieties can add an unexpected dimension to your snack.

- Presentation matters, even for small bites: Don't underestimate the power of a beautiful plate. Arrange your fruit and nut butter creations on a colorful platter, drizzle with honey or sprinkle with nuts and seeds for extra visual appeal. Make your snack time a feast for the eyes as well as the taste buds.

- Embrace the leftovers, even if there are none: This snack is so good, leftovers might be a rare occurrence. But if you do have some, fear not! Store them in an airtight container in the fridge and enjoy them as a second mini-snack later in the day.

- Make it your own: The beauty of this snack is its adaptability. Add a sprinkle of cinnamon to your apple slices, drizzle some honey on your mangoes, or toss your berries in a touch of coconut flakes. Experiment, innovate, and create your own signature fruit and nut butter masterpieces.

Remember, fruits with nut butter are not just a snack; they're an experience. Transform your snack time into a celebration of vibrant flavors, textures, and mindful well-being. Make your kitchen a creative canvas, your imagination your culinary guide, and every bite a testament to your love for simple pleasures and natural goodness.

Beyond the Plate: Embracing the Versatility of Fruits with Nut Butter

While the classic fruit and nut butter pairing shines on its own, its versatility shines even brighter when you move beyond the plate. Think of this dynamic duo as your culinary springboard, launching you into a world of creative and delicious snacking possibilities. Here are some beyond-the-plate adventures to awaken your inner culinary explorer:

- Smoothie Symphony: Blend sliced banana and almond butter with almond milk for a creamy and comforting smoothie. Play with different fruits and nut butter combinations, adding spinach for an extra nutritional boost or a teaspoon of raw cacao for a chocolatey twist.

- Yogurt Parfait Power: Layer Greek yogurt with your favorite sliced fruits and dollops of nut butter. Sprinkle with granola, chia seeds, or chopped nuts for added texture and flavor. This protein-packed parfait is a breakfast champion or a satisfying afternoon snack.

- Dipping Delight: Turn your snack into a social event! Slice a variety of fruits like apples, pears, grapes, and strawberries. Arrange them on a platter with different types of nut butter, and let everyone dip and enjoy. This interactive fun is perfect for parties or family gatherings.

- Baked Bliss: Turn fruit and nut butter into a warm and comforting treat. Spread nut butter on whole-wheat tortillas or pita bread, top with sliced apples or pears, and bake until golden brown. Drizzle with honey or sprinkle with cinnamon for an extra flavor punch.

- Overnight Oats Odyssey: Combine rolled oats, chia seeds, your favorite milk, and a teaspoon of nut butter in a jar. Top with sliced fruit and refrigerate overnight. In the morning, you'll have a ready-to-go, protein-packed breakfast that's full of flavor and texture.

- Energy Bites Explosion: Pulse chopped fruits, nut butter, oats, and a touch of honey in a food processor until a sticky dough forms. Roll into bite-sized balls and refrigerate. These nutrient-packed energy bites are the perfect on-the-go snack to keep your energy levels soaring.

Remember, the possibilities with fruits and nut butter are endless. Don't be afraid to experiment, get creative, and let your culinary imagination run wild. From simple slices to smoothie symphonies, this dynamic duo is your guide to a world of delicious, healthy, and endlessly satisfying snacking adventures. So, embrace the versatility, unleash your inner culinary artist, and create snack time memories that nourish your body and tantalize your taste buds.

Bonus Tip: When choosing nut butter, look for natural varieties with minimal added sugars or oils. Opt for organic options whenever possible to maximize the nutritional benefits and support sustainable farming practices.

Happy snacking and happy living!

Yogurt with Berries and Granola: Sweet and Nutritious

Beyond the Bowl: Unveiling the Symphony of Flavor and Texture in Yogurt with Berries and Granola - A Celebration of Sweetness and Nutritious Goodness

Forget the processed snacks and sugary treats. Ditch the guilt and embrace the joy. Your path to a vibrant, flavor-forward, and health-conscious snacking experience takes a refreshingly simple turn with the classic, yet endlessly customizable, combination of yogurt with berries and granola. Imagine, not settling for a monotonous nibble, but savoring a creamy and tart dance, punctuated by the satisfying crunch of toasted oats and seeds, all nestled in a symphony of textures and flavors that ignite your senses and nourish your body. Picture, not wrestling with hunger pangs or afternoon slumps, but enjoying a snack that keeps you feeling satisfied and energized, leaving you with a smile on your face and a glow of well-being radiating from within. Welcome to the world where yogurt with berries and granola become your snacktime champions, your kitchen a playground of possibilities, and every bite a celebration of simple ingredients, culinary creativity, and effortless well-being.

Why does this seemingly simple concoction hold the key to unlocking a winning snacktime experience? Here's the delicious breakdown:

- Sweet and Tart Tango: Ditch the one-dimensional flavor profiles. This dynamic trio offers a delightful interplay of sweetness and tartness. The natural sugars in berries burst on your tongue, while the creamy tang of yogurt creates a harmonious balance. Every bite is a flavor adventure, keeping your taste buds engaged and your snack routine exciting.

- Texture Symphony: One bowl does not equal boring! This combination embraces contrasting textures. The smooth creaminess of yogurt dances with the satisfying crunch of granola, while the juicy pop of berries adds a playful dimension. Each spoonful becomes a textural experience, keeping your senses entertained and making snacking more than just fuel.

- Nutrient Powerhouse: This snack packs a nutritional punch! Yogurt is a fantastic source of protein and calcium, essential for building and maintaining strong bones. Berries are bursting with vitamins, minerals, and antioxidants, protecting your cells and boosting your overall health. Granola, when chosen wisely, offers healthy fats, fiber, and even additional protein, making this snack a well-rounded nutritional champion.

- Convenience and Versatility: This snack is your anytime, anywhere companion. No elaborate preparation or fancy equipment needed! Grab a container of yogurt, sprinkle on some granola, top with your favorite berries, and voila – a delicious and nourishing snack ready in seconds. Whether you're on the go, at work, or relaxing at home, this dynamic trio has your back (and your stomach) covered.

- Mindful and Joyful Experience: This snack is not just about refueling; it's about pleasure. Savor the creamy coolness of the yogurt, the burst of berry sweetness, and the satisfying crunch of the granola. Appreciate the interplay of textures and flavors, and transform your snack break into a mini-ritual of self-care and joy.

Crafting Your Personal Yogurt with Berries and Granola Masterpiece:

- Choose your flavor adventure: Do you crave the classic sweetness of strawberries, or are you dreaming of a tart cherry explosion? Explore different berry and yogurt combinations, finding pairings that tantalize your taste buds and spark your culinary curiosity. Don't forget tropical options like mango or pineapple for a taste of sunshine!

- Get creative with textures: Go beyond the expected! Opt for Greek yogurt for a thicker and more protein-rich base, or try kefir for a tangy probiotic boost. Play with different granola varieties: add nuts and seeds for extra crunch, choose a chocolate drizzle for a touch of indulgence, or explore homemade options for complete control over the ingredients.

- Presentation matters, even for small bites: Don't underestimate the power of a beautiful bowl. Layer your yogurt, berries, and granola in a visually appealing way, drizzle with honey or chia seeds for added visual interest. Make your snack time a feast for the eyes as well as the taste buds.

- Embrace the leftovers, even if there are none: This snack is so good, leftovers might be a rare occurrence. But if you do have some, fear not! Store them in an airtight container in the fridge and enjoy them as a second mini-snack later in the day, or add them to smoothies or overnight oats for extra flavor and texture.

- Make it your own: The beauty of this snack is its adaptability. Add a sprinkle of cinnamon to your berries, whip in a spoonful of nut butter to your yogurt, or drizzle with a touch of maple syrup for extra sweetness. Experiment, innovate, and create your own signature yogurt with berries and granola masterpieces.

Remember, yogurt with berries and granola is not just a snack; it's an experience. Transform your snack time into a celebration of vibrant flavors, textures, and mindful well-being. Make your kitchen a creative canvas, your imagination your culinary guide, and every bite a testament to your love for simple pleasures and natural goodness. Embrace the versatility, unleash your inner culinary artist, and create snack time memories that nourish your body and tantalize your taste buds.

Beyond the Bowl: Unleashing the Full Potential of Your Snack Trio

While the classic yogurt, berries, and granola combination shines on its own, its potential extends far beyond the confines of a bowl. Think of this dynamic trio as your culinary springboard, launching you into a world of creative and refreshing snacking possibilities. Here are some beyond-the-bowl adventures to awaken your inner culinary explorer:

- Frozen Yogurt Bliss: Blend your favorite yogurt with berries and a touch of honey until smooth. Pour into popsicle molds or small paper cups and freeze for a healthy and refreshing frozen treat. Customize with different berry combinations, add a granola layer for extra texture, or drizzle with melted chocolate for a decadent twist.

- Smoothie Symphony: Transform your snack into a creamy and portable masterpiece. Blend yogurt, berries, a frozen banana, and your favorite milk until smooth. Add spinach or chia seeds for an extra nutritional boost, or use almond milk for a dairy-free option. This protein-packed smoothie is a breakfast champion or a satisfying afternoon pick-me-up.

- Overnight Oats Odyssey: Combine rolled oats, chia seeds, your favorite milk, and a spoonful of yogurt in a jar. Add a layer of mashed berries and refrigerate overnight. In the morning, you'll have a ready-to-go, protein-packed breakfast that's full of flavor and texture. Play with different berry combinations, sprinkle on granola for extra crunch, or drizzle with honey for added sweetness.

- Baked Bliss: Turn your snack into a warm and comforting treat. Spread yogurt on whole-wheat tortillas or pita bread, top with sliced berries and a sprinkle of granola. Bake until golden brown and enjoy a healthy and satisfying snack with a hint of sweetness. Try different berry toppings, drizzle with melted cinnamon for warmth, or experiment with savory versions using vegetables and herbs.

- Parfait Power: Layer crumbled cookies or graham crackers with yogurt, berries, and granola in a tall glass. Drizzle with honey or maple syrup for extra sweetness. This layered treat is perfect for satisfying your sweet tooth while packing in nutrients and healthy fats. Get creative with your layers, add a dollop of whipped cream for indulgence, or use different yogurt flavors for additional variety.

Remember, the possibilities with yogurt, berries, and granola are endless. Don't be afraid to experiment, get creative, and let your culinary imagination run wild. From simple bowls to smoothie symphonies, this dynamic trio is your guide to a world of delicious, healthy, and endlessly satisfying snacking adventures. So, embrace the versatility, unleash your inner culinary artist, and create snacktime memories that nourish your body and tantalize your taste buds.

Bonus Tip: When choosing yogurt, opt for plain, unsweetened varieties and control the sweetness yourself with natural sources like berries or honey. Look for granola with minimal added sugars and oils, focusing on options with nuts, seeds, and whole grains for maximum nutritional value.

Happy snacking and happy living!

Vegetable Sticks with Hummus: Fiber and Protein for Sustained Energy

Beyond the Ranch: Unveiling the Vibrant Symphony of Flavor and Nutritious Goodness in Vegetable Sticks with Hummus - A Celebration of Crunch and Cream

Forget the limp lettuce and greasy chips. Ditch the sugary dips and processed snacks. Your path to a vibrant, flavor-forward, and health-conscious snacking experience takes a refreshingly simple turn with the dynamic duo of vegetable sticks with hummus. Imagine, not settling for a monotonous nibble, but savoring a symphony of fresh and crisp textures punctuated by the creamy richness of hummus, all bursting with the goodness of colorful vegetables. Picture, not wrestling with hunger pangs or afternoon slumps, but enjoying a snack that keeps you feeling satisfied and energized, leaving you with a smile on your face and a glow of well-being radiating from within. Welcome to the world where vegetable sticks with hummus become your snacktime champions, your kitchen a playground of crunchy possibilities, and every bite a celebration of nature's bounty, culinary creativity, and effortless well-being.

Why does this seemingly simple combination hold the key to unlocking a winning snacktime experience? Here's the delicious breakdown:

- Crunch and Cream Tango: Ditch the one-dimensional textures. This dynamic duo offers a delightful interplay of satisfying crunch and creamy smoothness. The crisp snap of fresh vegetables creates a playful contrast to the richness of hummus, keeping your senses engaged and your taste buds entertained. Each bite becomes a textural adventure, making snacking more than just fuel.

- Fiber and Protein Powerhouse: One tray does not equal empty calories! This combination packs a nutritious punch. Vegetables are bursting with fiber, essential for digestive health and keeping you feeling full. Hummus, made from chickpeas, offers a generous dose of protein, key for building and maintaining muscle mass. Together, they create a satiating snack that keeps hunger at bay and fuels your energy levels throughout the day.

- Vitamin and Mineral Bounty: This snack is a rainbow of well-being! Different vegetables offer a diverse range of vitamins, minerals, and antioxidants, protecting your cells and boosting your overall health. Hummus, with its tahini and olive oil base, adds additional nutrients like calcium, iron, and healthy fats. Every bite becomes a journey through the land of well-being, nourishing your body with every flavorful crunch.

- Convenience and Versatility: This snack is your anytime, anywhere companion. No elaborate preparation or fancy equipment needed! Wash and cut your vegetables, grab a tub of hummus, and voila – a delicious and nourishing snack ready in seconds. Whether you're on the go, at work, or relaxing at home, this dynamic duo has your back (and your stomach) covered.

- Mindful and Joyful Experience: This snack is not just about refueling; it's about pleasure. Savor the fresh snap of the vegetables, the creamy richness of the hummus, the interplay of textures and flavors. Appreciate the vibrant colors and the simple joy of nourishing your body. Transform your snack break into a mini-ritual of self-care and joy, a mindful moment amidst the busy day.

Crafting Your Personal Vegetable Stick and Hummus Masterpiece:

- Choose your crunchy symphony: Do you crave the classic coolness of cucumber sticks, or are you dreaming of a fiery bell pepper tango? Explore different vegetable options, finding combinations that tantalize your taste buds and ignite your culinary curiosity. Don't forget seasonal favorites like baby carrots, celery stalks, or snap peas for added variety.

- Get creative with hummus: Go beyond the expected! Choose flavors that compliment your chosen vegetables. Garlic hummus adds a spicy kick to cucumber sticks, while roasted red pepper hummus pairs beautifully with bell peppers. Explore homemade options if you feel adventurous, or experiment with flavored varieties like jalapeno or beetroot for a unique twist.

- Presentation matters, even for small bites: Don't underestimate the power of a beautiful platter. Arrange your vegetable sticks in a visually appealing way, contrasting colors and textures for added interest. Dip your hummus in a bowl or dollop it onto the platter for a more interactive experience. Make your snack time a feast for the eyes as well as the taste buds.

- Embrace the leftovers, even if there are none: This snack is so good, leftovers might be a rare occurrence. But if you do have some, fear not! Store leftover vegetables in an airtight container in the fridge and hummus in its original container. Enjoy them as another mini-snack later in the day, add them to salads or wraps, or experiment with creative leftovers recipes like veggie fritters or hummus quesadillas.

- Make it your own: The beauty of this snack is its adaptability. Add a sprinkle of your favorite spice blend to your hummus, drizzle with olive oil or lemon juice for extra flavor, or try different dipping options like guacamole or pesto for a global twist. Experiment, innovate, and create your own signature vegetable stick and hummus masterpieces.

Remember, vegetable sticks with hummus are not just a snack they're an experience. Transform your snack time into a celebration of vibrant textures, flavors, and mindful well-being. Make your kitchen a creative canvas, your imagination your culinary guide, and every bite a testament to your love for simple pleasures and natural goodness. Embrace the versatility, unleash your inner culinary artist, and create snack time memories that nourish your body and tantalize your taste buds.

Beyond the Tray: Unleashing the Full Potential of Your Crunchy and Creamy Duo

While the classic vegetable sticks and hummus combination shines on its own, its potential extends far beyond the confines of a tray. Think of this dynamic duo as your culinary springboard, launching you into a world of creative and refreshing snacking possibilities. Here are some beyond-the-tray adventures to awaken your inner culinary explorer:

- Hummus Smoothie Powerhouse: Blend hummus with your favorite yogurt, spinach, and a touch of honey for a creamy and protein-packed smoothie. Add slices of banana or berries for sweetness and texture, or toss in a handful of leafy greens for an extra nutrient boost. This protein-rich smoothie is a breakfast champion or a satisfying afternoon pick-me-up.

- Snack Bowl Odyssey: Combine chopped vegetables, whole-grain crackers, and crumbled feta cheese in a bowl. Top with dollops of hummus and drizzle with olive oil and lemon juice for a satisfying and flavorful snack. Play with different vegetable and cracker combinations, add a sprinkle of nuts or seeds for extra crunch, or experiment with different protein options like chicken breast or hard-boiled eggs.

- Stuffed Pepper Symphony: Slice bell peppers in half and roast them until tender. Fill them with hummus, chopped vegetables, and crumbled tofu or chickpeas for a warm and satisfying snack. This protein-packed option is perfect for a light lunch or a post-workout treat. Get creative with your fillings, add avocado slices for creaminess, or try different hummus flavors for a unique twist.

- Hummus Toast Extravaganza: Toast whole-wheat bread or pita bread and spread it with hummus. Top with your favorite vegetable combinations, a sprinkle of herbs, and a drizzle of olive oil or balsamic vinegar for a healthy and flavorful open-faced sandwich. Experiment with different toppings like roasted tomatoes, grilled eggplant, or sliced mushrooms for endless possibilities.

- Veggie Fritter Fun: Combine leftover chopped vegetables with mashed chickpeas, herbs, and spices. Form into patties and pan-fry or bake until golden brown. Serve with hummus for a healthy and delicious appetizer or snack. Play with different spices and herbs to create your own signature fritter flavors, or add grated cheese or chopped nuts for extra texture.

Remember, the possibilities with vegetable sticks and hummus are endless. Don't be afraid to experiment, get creative, and let your culinary imagination run wild. From simple trays to smoothie symphonies, this dynamic duo is your guide to a world of delicious, healthy, and endlessly satisfying snacking adventures. So, embrace the versatility, unleash your inner culinary artist, and create snacktime memories that nourish your body and tantalize your taste buds.

Bonus Tip: When choosing hummus, opt for natural varieties with minimal added fats and oils. Look for versions made with tahini and olive oil for added nutrients and flavor. Remember, fresh vegetables are your friends! So choose seasonal options whenever possible for maximum flavor and nutritional value.

Happy snacking and happy living!

Homemade Trail Mix: Customize Your Perfect Snack Blend

Beyond the Grocery Aisle: Unleashing the Creativity and Savory Symphony of Homemade Trail Mix - A Celebration of Customized Fuel and Flavor

Forget the same-old, processed bags hiding a bland mix of stale nuts and dusty raisins. Ditch the artificial flavors and hidden sugars masquerading as healthy snacks. Your path to a vibrant, customizable, and flavor-forward experience takes a delightful turn with the world of homemade trail mix. Imagine, not settling for a monotonous nibble, but crafting your own symphony of textures, tastes, and nutrients, tailored to your unique cravings and dietary needs. Picture, not succumbing to hunger pangs or afternoon slumps, but fueling your body and delighting your taste buds with a personalized concoction that keeps you feeling satisfied and energized, leaving you with a smile on your face and a sense of culinary accomplishment. Welcome to the world where homemade trail mix becomes your snacktime champion, your pantry a playground of possibilities, and every handful a celebration of creativity, mindful munching, and well-being.

Why does this seemingly simple blend hold the key to unlocking a winning snacktime experience? Here's the delicious breakdown:

- Customizable Symphony: One mix does not equal boring! This blank canvas welcomes endless creativity. Crave the creamy richness of cashews alongside the tart pop of dried cranberries? Longing for the salty satisfaction of roasted chickpeas paired with the sweetness of banana chips? Go for it! Your trail mix, your rules. Explore different ingredients, flavors, and textures, finding combinations that tantalize your taste buds and ignite your culinary curiosity.

- Nutrient Powerhouse: This snack packs a personalized punch! Nuts offer healthy fats and protein, while dried fruits burst with vitamins, minerals, and antioxidants. Seeds add fiber and essential nutrients, while dark chocolate can even provide health benefits in moderation. Tailor your mix to your dietary needs and preferences, creating a snack that nourishes your body while satisfying your cravings.

- Convenience and Versatility: This snack travels anywhere with you. No fancy equipment or elaborate preparation needed! Toss your chosen ingredients in a container, and voila – a delicious and nourishing snack ready in seconds. Whether you're on the go, at work, or relaxing at home, your personalized trail mix has your back (and your stomach) covered.

- Mindful and Joyful Experience: This snack is not just about refueling; it's about the experience. Savor the contrasting textures of crunchy nuts and chewy fruits, the interplay of sweet and salty flavors, the vibrant colors pleasing your eyes. Appreciate the act of creating your own blend, savoring each bite with the knowledge that you crafted this for yourself. Transform your snack break into a mini-ritual of self-care and joy, a mindful moment amidst the busy day.

Crafting Your Masterpiece Trail Mix:

- Choose your flavor adventure: Do you crave a tropical escape with mango chunks and coconut flakes, or are you dreaming of a spicy fiesta with roasted chickpeas and chili flakes? Explore different ingredient categories: nuts, seeds, dried fruits, chocolate, and even savory options like roasted chickpeas or seaweed snacks. Mix and match, play with proportions, and find your perfect flavor balance.

- Get creative with textures: Go beyond the expected! Roast your nuts for extra depth of flavor, slice your dried fruits for smaller bites, or crush your favorite dark chocolate into pieces for a decadent surprise. Play with shapes, sizes, and textures to create a mix that's not just delicious, but also visually appealing.

- Presentation matters, even for small bites: Don't underestimate the power of a beautiful container. Choose a reusable jar or airtight container with a secure lid. Layer your ingredients to create visual interest, or sprinkle on a few edible flowers for a touch of whimsy. Make your snack time a feast for the eyes as well as the taste buds.

- Embrace the leftovers, even if there are none: This snack is so good, leftovers might be a rare occurrence. But if you do have some, fear not! Store them in an airtight container in the fridge to preserve freshness. Enjoy them as another mini-snack later in the day, add them to your yogurt or oatmeal for extra flavor and texture, or sprinkle them on a salad for a crunchy garnish.

- Make it your own: The beauty of this snack is its adaptability. Add a sprinkle of your favorite spice blend to your nuts, drizzle with honey or melted chocolate for extra sweetness, or toss in a handful of shredded coconut for a tropical twist. Experiment, innovate, and create your own signature trail mix masterpieces.

Remember, homemade trail mix is not just a snack; it's an experience. Transform your snack time into a celebration of personalized flavors, textures, and mindful well-being. Make your pantry a creative canvas, your imagination your culinary guide, and every handful a testament to your love for simple pleasures and personalized well-being. Embrace the versatility, unleash your inner culinary artist, and create snacktime memories that nourish your body and tantalize your taste buds.

Beyond the Bowl: Unleashing the Full Potential of Your Customized Blend

While the classic handful enjoyed straight from the container is a delightful experience in itself, your homemade trail mix holds the potential for adventures that extend far beyond the confines of the bowl. Think of this dynamic blend as your culinary springboard, launching you into a world of creative and refreshing snacking possibilities. Here are some beyond-the-bowl adventures to awaken your inner culinary explorer:

- Energy Bites Bliss: Pulse your favorite trail mix ingredients in a food processor until a sticky dough forms. Roll into bite-sized balls and refrigerate. These nutrient-packed energy bites are perfect for pre-workout fuel, an afternoon pick-me-up, or a satisfying dessert alternative. Play with different ingredients, add oats for extra texture, or drizzle with melted chocolate for a decadent touch.

- Parfait Powerhouse: Layer yogurt, crumbled cookies or granola, and your trail mix in a tall glass. Drizzle with honey or maple syrup for extra sweetness. This layered treat is perfect for a quick and filling breakfast or a snack that satisfies both your sweet tooth and your desire for healthy fats and protein. Get creative with your layers, add a dollop of whipped cream for indulgence, or use different yogurt flavors for additional variety.

- Salad Sensation: Sprinkle your trail mix on top of your favorite salad for a burst of texture, flavor, and nutrients. Nuts add healthy fats, seeds provide fiber and essential minerals, while dried fruits offer a touch of sweetness. This simple sprinkle instantly elevates your salad from a side dish to a satisfying main course. Experiment with different salad components, add a protein like grilled chicken or tofu, and drizzle with a flavorful dressing for a complete and delicious meal.

- Dip and Crunch Extravaganza: Use your trail mix as a dip for fresh fruit slices like apple, pear, or banana. The creamy richness of nuts and the natural sweetness of dried fruits complement the fresh flavors of the fruit, creating a satisfying and healthy snacking experience. Try different nut and fruit combinations, experiment with savory dips like hummus or guacamole, or use whole-grain crackers or rice cakes for a heartier option.

- Baked Bliss: Turn your trail mix into a warm and comforting treat. Spread nut butter on whole-wheat tortillas or pita bread, top with your favorite trail mix blend, and bake until golden brown. Drizzle with honey or sprinkle with cinnamon for extra warmth and flavor. This protein-packed treat is perfect for a light lunch, a post-workout snack, or a satisfying dessert alternative. Play with different nut butter and trail mix combinations, add sliced banana or apples for additional moisture, or get creative with savory options like pesto and roasted vegetables.

Remember, the possibilities with homemade trail mix are endless. Don't be afraid to experiment, get creative, and let your culinary imagination run wild. From simple handfuls to energy bites bliss, this customizable blend is your guide to a world of delicious, healthy, and endlessly satisfying snacking adventures. So, embrace the versatility, unleash your inner culinary artist, and create snacktime memories that nourish your body and tantalize your taste buds.

Bonus Tip: When choosing ingredients for your trail mix, opt for unsalted and unsweetened options whenever possible. Look for nuts and seeds with minimal added oils or spices, and choose dried fruits without added sugars or preservatives. Remember, fresh is best! Opt for in-season fruits whenever possible for maximum flavor and nutritional value.

Happy snacking and happy living!

Part 3: Putting it All Together: Combining Workout and Recipes for Success

Chapter 11: Planning Your Week: Workouts and Meals in Harmony

Scheduling Workouts: Finding Time for Fitness in Your Busy Life

Chapter 11: Planning Your Week: Workouts and Meals in Harmony

Scheduling Workouts: Finding Time for Fitness in Your Busy Life

We've talked about the benefits of easy workouts and delicious, healthy recipes for those over 60. But how do you actually fit it all into your already-packed schedule? Let's face it, life gets busy, and carving out time for self-care, especially exercise, can feel like trying to squeeze water out of a stone. Worry not, my fellow fitness and food enthusiasts! This chapter is all about conquering the scheduling beast and weaving movement and meals into your daily tapestry with grace and efficiency.

Know Your Why:

Before you dive into calendar battles, revisit your "why." What motivates you to move your body and nourish it with goodness? Is it improved energy levels, sharper focus, stronger muscles, or simply the joy of feeling good in your own skin? Re-igniting your purpose will provide the fuel to power through scheduling hurdles.

Assessing Your Landscape:

Take a realistic inventory of your week. Map out your commitments – work, family, social obligations, even those Netflix marathons! Be honest about your energy levels and free time blocks. Identify potential workout windows, even if they're just 15-minute slivers between errands. Remember, consistency is key – small, regular doses of movement are far more beneficial than sporadic bursts of exertion.

Embrace Micro-Workouts:

Think outside the gym box! Micro-workouts are your secret weapon for busy bees. Sneak in squats while brushing your teeth, lunge during commercial breaks, or take the stairs instead of the elevator. Every little movement counts and adds up throughout the day. Aim for at least 3-5 micro-workouts daily, each lasting 5-10 minutes. You'll be surprised at how quickly those minutes morph into a significant energy boost and calorie burn.

Schedule Like a Pro:

Treat your workouts like VIP appointments. Block out dedicated time slots in your calendar, and treat them with the same respect you would a doctor's appointment. This makes your commitment visible and less likely to be bumped off the list by less important tasks. Bonus points for setting recurring appointments, creating a consistent routine that becomes as automatic as brushing your teeth.

Find Your Fitness Family:

Having a workout buddy or joining a group fitness class can be a game-changer. The social aspect adds a layer of fun and accountability, making it harder to skip sessions. Plus, group workouts can offer variety and motivation, pushing you beyond your comfort zone in a supportive environment.

Think Beyond the Gym:

Remember, exercise doesn't have to be confined to a gym. Embrace the outdoors! Take a brisk walk in the park, do some gardening yoga in your backyard, or join a lunchtime dance class. Explore activities you enjoy – swimming, dancing, hiking – and turn them into your personalized fitness playground.

Master the Art of Multitasking:

Combine chores with movement. Listen to audiobooks or podcasts while walking or gardening. Turn running errands into mini fitness adventures – park further away and walk, take the stairs whenever possible. Every step counts, and you'll get things done while breaking a sweat.

Embrace Morning Magic:

Mornings can be a goldmine for exercise. Waking up just 30 minutes earlier can unlock a prime fitness window before the day's whirlwind takes hold. A morning workout jumpstarts your metabolism, sets a positive tone for the day, and leaves you feeling energized and accomplished.

Listen to Your Body:

Remember, scheduling isn't a rigid dictatorship. Be flexible and listen to your body's needs. If you're feeling drained, skip the scheduled workout and prioritize rest. Listen to your energy levels and adjust your plan accordingly. Consistency is key, but so is self-compassion.

Embrace Technology:

Apps and wearable devices can be your digital cheerleaders. Use workout apps to find new routines, track your progress, and stay motivated. Fitness trackers can monitor your steps, heart rate, and overall activity levels, providing valuable data and a sense of accomplishment.

Reward Yourself:

Celebrate your wins! Hitting your weekly workout goals deserves a pat on the back. Treat yourself to a massage, a new workout outfit, or a night out with friends. Positive reinforcement keeps you motivated and on track.

Remember, finding time for fitness is a journey, not a destination. Be patient, experiment, and have fun! Embrace the flexibility of micro-workouts, schedule strategically, and most importantly, listen to your body. With dedication and a little creativity, you can weave movement seamlessly into the tapestry of your life, reaping the rewards of feeling fitter, healthier, and happier than ever before.

Bonus Tips:

Prepare for success: Set out your workout clothes the night before to avoid morning procrastination.

Pack a gym bag full of essentials to avoid scrambling before workouts. Include comfy shoes, breathable clothes, a water bottle, a light towel, and maybe a healthy snack for after.

Get creative with your space: Don't have a gym membership or fancy equipment? No worries! A yoga mat, resistance bands, or even a sturdy chair can become your home gym. Utilize online workout channels for guided routines, or get inspired by YouTube fitness tutorials.

Team up with technology: Utilize online booking platforms to schedule fitness classes at convenient times and locations. Invest in a fitness tracker or smartwatch to monitor your progress and stay motivated. Download apps for interval timers, music playlists, or guided meditations for post-workout relaxation.

Think beyond the clock: Remember, exercise isn't just about structured workouts. Take the stairs instead of the elevator, park further away and walk, do lunges while waiting for the kettle to boil – every little movement counts. Integrate activity into your daily routine throughout the day.

Don't be afraid to ask for help: Seeking support from a personal trainer or fitness coach can be a game-changer. They can design personalized workout plans, provide guidance on form and technique, and offer valuable motivation and accountability.

Embrace flexibility: Life happens, and schedules shift. Don't beat yourself up if you miss a workout or two. Be flexible and adjust your plan as needed. Remember, consistency is key, but progress, not perfection, is the ultimate goal.

Make it fun!: Choose activities you genuinely enjoy. Dance to your favorite music, go for a scenic bike ride, join a fun group fitness class, or explore a new sport. When exercise feels like play, you're more likely to stick with it and reap the long-term benefits.

Celebrate success: Track your progress, be proud of your achievements, and reward yourself for reaching milestones. A new workout outfit, a relaxing spa day, or a delicious healthy meal can be your way of acknowledging your commitment and motivating yourself to keep going.

Remember, incorporating fitness into your busy life is a journey, not a sprint. Be kind to yourself, embrace flexibility, and celebrate every step you take towards a healthier, happier you. With a little planning, creativity, and the right mindset, you can weave movement seamlessly into the tapestry of your life and unlock the joy of feeling fit and vibrant at any age.

Now go forth, conquer your schedule, and embrace the amazing journey of building a life infused with movement, healthy nourishment, and endless possibilities!

Meal Planning Made Easy: Grocery Shopping with Efficiency

Meal Planning Made Easy: Grocery Shopping with Efficiency

Conquering your workout schedule feels like a triumph, but the battle isn't over! Next comes the seemingly daunting task of grocery shopping. Visions of overflowing carts, impulsive buys, and forgotten ingredients dance in your head. Fear not, my fellow food enthusiasts! This chapter unlocks the secrets of meal planning made easy, transforming grocery shopping into an efficient, organized, and surprisingly enjoyable experience.

Embrace the Magic of Meal Planning:

Think of meal planning as your food fairy godmother, orchestrating delicious, healthy meals with minimal stress. By mapping out your weekly menu, you'll avoid last-minute scrambles, combat food waste, and ensure your fridge is stocked with nutritious goodness. Plus, it saves you time (and money!) by minimizing impulsive purchases during rushed supermarket adventures.

Start with a Foundation:

1. Assess your needs: Consider your dietary preferences, allergies, and any family restrictions. Prioritize fruits, vegetables, whole grains, and lean protein sources.

2. Inventory your pantry and fridge: Take stock of existing ingredients to avoid duplication and waste. Plan meals around what you already have, incorporating those items first.

3. Choose your recipes: Select simple, healthy recipes that fit your schedule and culinary skills. Online recipe platforms, cookbooks, and even meal planning apps can be your inspiration gurus.

4. Plan for leftovers: Leftovers are your secret weapon! Double up on certain meals and repurpose them for lunches or quick dinners later in the week.

Craft Your Shopping List:

1. Categorize and conquer: Make a master list, grouping items by section (dairy, produce, pantry staples, etc.) This streamlines your shopping journey and minimizes aisle-backtracking.

2. Quantify with clarity: Don't be vague. List specific quantities for each ingredient, avoiding ambiguous phrases like "a few" or "some." Precision equals efficiency!

3. Factor in snacks: Don't forget healthy snacks! Include fruits, vegetables, nuts, yogurt, or homemade trail mix to keep hunger pangs at bay.

4. Price matters: Check weekly flyers and coupons to maximize your budget. Consider store brands for staples and compare prices before reaching for fancy labels.

Mastering the Grocery Game:

1. Shop with a full stomach: Hunger pangs lead to impulse buys. A pre-shopping snack keeps your cravings in check and your wallet thanking you.

2. Stick to your list: It's your roadmap to efficiency. Resist the siren song of tempting side aisles and focus on your pre-planned ingredients.

3. Embrace bulk buying: If you have the storage space, buying in bulk can save money on frequently used staples like rice, beans, or oatmeal. Just be mindful of expiration dates and portion control.

4. Don't fear frozen: Frozen fruits and vegetables are often flash-frozen at peak ripeness, locking in nutrients and flavor. They're also budget-friendly and convenient – a pantry must-have for busy schedules.

5. Befriend the produce section: Prioritize fresh fruits and vegetables, but don't shy away from pre-washed or pre-chopped options for time-saving convenience.

6. Check those expiration dates: Be vigilant! Expired items are a waste of money and potentially harmful. Double-check dates before adding anything to your cart.

7. Pack your reusable bags: Be eco-conscious and ditch the plastic. Reusable bags are convenient, sturdy, and help reduce environmental impact.

Beyond the Cart:

1. Organize your groceries: Upon arrival home, unpack and store your purchases strategically. Group similar items together, label leftovers for clear identification, and place high-priority ingredients within easy reach.

2. Clean and prep: Wash fruits and vegetables, pre-chop some vegetables for stir-fries or salads, and portion out ingredients for upcoming meals. This simplifies daily cooking and saves precious time later.

3. Utilize storage containers: Airtight containers keep your food fresh and prevent spoilage. Utilize reusable portion-control containers for lunches or snacks to avoid overeating.

4. Embrace batch cooking: Cook larger batches of certain dishes (soups, stews, chili) and freeze or store in airtight containers for quick and healthy meals throughout the week.

Remember, meal planning and grocery shopping are skills that improve with practice. Don't be discouraged by minor hiccups or forgotten ingredients. Embrace the learning process, adapt your strategies, and celebrate your wins, however small they may seem. With dedication and a bit of planning, you'll transform yourself into a grocery-shopping ninja, wielding efficiency and healthy eating like your secret superpowers.

So, go forth, brave warriors! Conquer your pantry, master the aisles, and unlock the joy of nourishing your body with delicious, healthy meals – all thanks to the magic of meal planning.

Batch Cooking: Prepare Healthy Meals in Advance for the Week

Batch Cooking: Prepare Healthy Meals in Advance for the Week

Conquering your workout schedule and mastering grocery shopping are impressive feats, but the quest for ultimate weeknight peace reaches its pinnacle with the art of batch cooking. Imagine: delicious, healthy meals readily available all week, without the evening scramble and takeout temptations. Sounds like a dream? It's not! Dive into this chapter and transform your kitchen into a haven of prepped perfection, leaving your future self infinitely grateful.

Why Batch Cooking is a Game-Changer:

- Save time and sanity: No more frantic dinner dashes after work. Prepping meals in advance liberates your evenings for relaxation, social activities, or, gasp, another workout!

- Boost health and budget: Batch cooking encourages healthy choices, as you're in control of ingredients and portion sizes. Plus, buying larger quantities often saves money compared to purchasing smaller amounts throughout the week.

- Reduce food waste: By pre-measuring and utilizing leftovers, you'll send less food to the compost bin, saving money and contributing to a more sustainable lifestyle.

- Enjoy variety and flavor: Batch cooking doesn't mean repetitive meals! Plan different dishes for each day, experiment with fresh ingredients, and freeze portions for future adventures in taste.

Mastering the Batch Cook:

1. Plan your meals: Choose recipes that lend themselves well to batching, like soups, stews, chili, pasta sauces, or casseroles. Consider dietary needs and preferences, incorporating variety and balance.

2. Prep day magic: Block out a dedicated time for batch cooking, perhaps a weekend afternoon. Gather all ingredients, pre-chop vegetables, measure spices, and cook larger batches. Utilize slow cookers or Instant Pots for added efficiency.

3. Portion perfect: Divide cooked meals into individual containers or bags, ensuring you have easy, grab-and-go options for the entire week. Label each container with the dish name and date to avoid fridge-spelunking confusion.

4. Storage solutions: Utilize airtight containers or freezer bags for optimal storage. Consider labeling frozen portions with expiry dates to ensure timely consumption.

5. Reheating like a pro: Thaw frozen meals overnight in the refrigerator or gently reheat in a microwave or on the stovetop. Avoid overcooking to preserve flavor and texture.

Beyond the Basics:

- Leftover love: Don't just reheat! Get creative with leftovers. Leftover chicken can become a salad topping, a stir-fry base, or pizza topping. Quinoa can be added to soups or stuffed into peppers. Think outside the fridge box!

- Soup swaps: Make a large pot of lentil soup and swap out toppings throughout the week for variety. Try crumbled feta and fresh herbs, crunchy croutons and Parmesan, or a dollop of pesto and a drizzle of balsamic vinegar.

- Breakfast prep: Batch cook oatmeal or muffins for quick, grab-and-go mornings. Overnight oats with berries and nuts offer a portable, protein-packed option.

- Snack smart: Pre-portioned fruits and vegetables, Greek yogurt parfaits with granola, or homemade trail mix offer healthy alternatives to processed snacks.

Embrace the Flexibility:

Life happens, and schedules shift. Don't get discouraged if you can't cook in advance every week. Even cooking one or two large batches can significantly reduce your weeknight cooking workload. Adapt your plan as needed, and celebrate every victory, big or small.

Remember, batch cooking is a journey, not a destination. Experiment, discover new recipes, and find what works best for you. The key is to find a process that fits your lifestyle and preferences, allowing you to enjoy healthy, delicious meals throughout the week without sacrificing precious time or sanity.

So, go forth, brave pioneers of prepped perfection! Conquer your fridge, embrace the batch, and unlock the joy of stress-free dinners and endless culinary possibilities. Your future self (and taste buds) will thank you!

Bonus Tip: Get the family involved! Assign tasks, delegate chopping, and turn batch cooking into a fun, collaborative activity. Bonding, laughter, and delicious meals? Batch cooking just keeps getting better!

Leftovers as Lunch: Repurpose Dinners for Delicious Midday Meals

Leftovers as Lunch: Repurpose Dinners for Delicious Midday Meals

Ah, the humble leftover. Often relegated to the back of the fridge and forgotten, these culinary castaways hold the potential for midday magic! In this chapter, we'll break the stigma surrounding leftovers and transform them into the stars of your lunchbox, showcasing their delicious potential and saving you time, money, and precious kitchen hours.

Why Leftovers Make Lunchtime Legends:

- Time-saving superstars: Say goodbye to rushed pre-lunch chaos! Leftovers offer instant nourishment, requiring minimal assembly and eliminating the need for frantic sandwich construction or microwaveable mysteries.

- Budget-savvy champions: Who needs takeout when you have a fridge full of culinary gold? Leftovers stretch your food budget further, preventing wasted ingredients and maximizing the life of every delicious purchase.

- Variety and flavor: Leftovers aren't monotonous! With a little creativity, they can morph into entirely new dishes, offering exciting flavor combinations and keeping your midday meals interesting.

- Sustainability heroes: Repurposing food is an eco-friendly act! By reducing food waste, you minimize your environmental impact and contribute to a more sustainable lifestyle.

Leftover Repurposing Magic:

- Dinner-to-salad transformation: Roast chicken becomes a protein-packed salad topping, roasted vegetables add vibrant color and texture, and leftover grains serve as a hearty base. Toss in some fresh greens, a drizzle of dressing, and voila, a gourmet salad without the gourmet price tag.

- Soup so good: Leftover stews, chili, or even roasted vegetables can be reborn as nourishing soups. Simply blend, add broth, customize with spices, and enjoy a steaming bowl of goodness that warms you from the inside out.

- Wraps and rolls on the go: Leftover shredded chicken or tofu gets a new lease on life in wraps or rolls. Add crunchy veggies, a touch of sauce, and wrap it up in a whole-wheat tortilla or rice paper for a portable, satisfying lunch.

- Frittatas and quiche champions: Leftover vegetables, cheese, and meats find a glorious second act in frittatas or quiches. Whip up a quick egg mixture, pour it over your leftover goodies, and bake for a protein-packed, customizable lunch that's perfect hot or cold.

- Sandwiches with sass: Don't settle for boring! Leftover pasta salad becomes a sandwich spread, roasted sweet potatoes transform into sweet and savory sandwich fillers, and grilled salmon or tofu can be reborn as the star of a gourmet open-faced creation.

Packing Your Leftover Lunchbox Wisdom:

- Storage is key: Invest in leak-proof containers and compartmentalized lunchboxes to prevent soggy disasters and keep your ingredients separate.

- Portion control matters: Divide leftovers into individual portions to avoid overeating and ensure lunch doesn't overshadow dinner.

- Temperature matters: Keep cold foods cold and hot foods hot. Use insulated lunch bags or ice packs for perishable items, and consider reheating options for heartier dishes.

- Spice it up!: Don't let leftovers get the "same old" blues. Add a squeeze of lemon, a sprinkle of fresh herbs, or a dollop of your favorite hot sauce to awaken flavors and keep your taste buds excited.

- Get creative!: Leftovers are a blank canvas for culinary adventures. Don't be afraid to experiment, mix and match flavors, and have fun with food!

Embrace the Leftover Revolution:

By viewing leftovers not as culinary castaways, but as delicious possibilities, you unlock a world of convenience, flavor, and resourcefulness. Leftovers empower you to eat well, save money, and reduce waste, all while saving precious time for the things that truly matter. So, the next time dinner comes to an end, remember, the real magic often begins the next day, disguised as a humble, yet delicious, leftover.

Bonus Tip: Get the family involved! Have leftover planning sessions, encourage creative lunchbox creations, and turn leftovers into a fun, collaborative culinary exploration.

Go forth, leftover champions! Embrace the repurpose, conquer the lunchbox, and unlock the full potential of your fridge's forgotten treasures. Remember, with a little imagination and a dash of creativity, leftovers can become the stars of your lunch show, nourishing your body and wallet in equal measure. Bon appétit!

Chapter 12: Adapting Your Plan: Listening to Your Body and Making Adjustments

Recognizing Rest Days: Importance of Recovery for Active Aging

Recognizing Rest Days: The Fuel Gauge for Active Aging

In the age-defying quest for fitness and health, it's easy to fall into the trap of "more is more." We push ourselves through workouts, feeling the exhilarating burn of activity, and relish the accomplishment of ticking another day off the exercise calendar. But just like a car engine thrives on regular oil changes and pit stops, our bodies, especially in the silver years, require mindful periods of rest and recuperation. Recognizing and embracing rest days isn't a sign of weakness or laziness; it's a crucial component of active aging, the secret sauce that unlocks sustained progress and long-term well-being.

Why Rest Matters More After 60:

With age, our bodies naturally experience physiological changes that impact recovery. Cell regeneration slows down, muscle tissue rebuilds at a slower pace, and hormonal fluctuations can affect energy levels. Pushing through these limitations without adequate rest can lead to a cascade of negative consequences:

- Overtraining Syndrome: This insidious condition arises from chronic overexertion. Symptoms like fatigue, decreased performance, persistent muscle soreness, and even insomnia can significantly derail your fitness journey.

- Increased Risk of Injuries: Overworked muscles and joints become vulnerable to strains, sprains, and even fractures.

Taking rest days allows for tissue repair and prevents these painful setbacks.

- Diminished Motivation: If you constantly feel drained and achy, your enthusiasm for exercise wanes. Rest days allow your body to replenish energy and reignite the spark of enjoyment in your active routine.

- Compromised Immune System: When your body is constantly in repair mode, its ability to fight off infections diminishes. Regular rest strengthens your immune system, keeping you healthy and ready to tackle your workouts with gusto.

Beyond Physical Benefits:

The importance of rest days extends far beyond just physical recuperation. When you give your body a break, you allow your mind and spirit to recharge too:

- Stress Reduction: Exercise itself can be a stress reliever, but pushing through exhaustion can have the opposite effect. Rest days provide a much-needed mental break, lowering cortisol levels and promoting feelings of calm and well-being.

- Improved Sleep Quality: Regular physical activity promotes better sleep, but overtraining can disrupt your sleep cycle, leaving you feeling even more fatigued. Rest days give your body a chance to wind down and prepare for restorative sleep.

- Enhanced Creativity and Focus: Physical exertion stimulates the brain, but constant activity can lead to mental fatigue and decreased cognitive function. Rest days allow for mental clarity, making you more productive and creative in other aspects of your life.

- Greater Appreciation for Movement: When you truly experience the benefits of rest, you return to your workouts with renewed appreciation for the joy of movement. This shift in perspective leads to a more sustainable and enjoyable approach to fitness.

Listening to Your Body's Cues:

So, how do you know when it's time to hit the brakes and prioritize rest? Your body will whisper the answer if you listen closely. Some telltale signs include:

- Persistent Muscle Soreness: Soreness from a tough workout is normal, but if it lingers for days or interferes with your daily activities, take a break.

- Decreased Performance: If you notice a sudden drop in your usual workout capacity, it's a sign that your body needs time to rebuild.

- Fatigue and Lack of Motivation: Feeling constantly drained and uninspired to exercise? Your body is likely pleading for a pause.

- Sleep Disturbances: Difficulty falling asleep, restless nights, or waking up feeling unrefreshed are often indicators of overtraining.

- Headaches and Irritability: These seemingly unrelated symptoms can also be signals of a body crying out for rest.

Making Rest Days Count:

Rest doesn't have to mean lying on the couch all day. Embrace active recovery strategies that promote healing and rejuvenation:

- Gentle stretching and yoga: These activities improve flexibility and blood flow while calming the mind and body.

- Walking in nature: Immersing yourself in the outdoors lowers stress levels and promotes a sense of peace.

- Swimming or water aerobics: The buoyancy of water reduces pressure on joints while providing a low-impact workout.

- Meditation or mindfulness practices: Quiet your mind and allow your body to unwind through deep breathing and relaxation techniques.

- Creative pursuits: Spend time on hobbies you enjoy, whether it's painting, writing, or playing music. These activities can relieve stress and spark joy.

Remember, rest days are not indulgences; they are investments in your long-term fitness journey. By incorporating them into your routine, you'll build a foundation for sustainable health and vibrant living, proving that active aging is not about pushing through pain, but about listening to your body and honoring its wisdom. So, embrace the stillness, let your muscles rebuild, and prepare to return to your workouts with renewed vigor and a spirit of playful joy. Remember, you're not running a race against time, but embarking on a beautiful dance with your body, one that celebrates movement, respects its limitations, and fuels a lifelong pursuit of well-being.

Bonus Tips for Active Rest:

- Schedule your rest days: Planning them in advance ensures you prioritize them and don't accidentally push yourself too hard.

- Listen to your intuition: Don't wait for your body to scream; if you feel a niggling doubt about pushing through, err on the side of caution and rest.

- Fuel your recovery: Eat nourishing meals rich in protein and healthy fats to provide your body with the building blocks it needs to repair and rebuild.

- Stay hydrated: Water is essential for muscle recovery and overall health. Make sure you drink plenty throughout the day, especially on rest days.

- Connect with loved ones: Social interaction and emotional support can be very restorative. Spend time with family and friends or join a social group focused on active aging.

- Celebrate your progress: Recognize the achievements of your body, not just on workout days, but also on rest days. Acknowledge the importance of giving yourself time to heal and replenish.

By incorporating these practices, you can transform your rest days from guilt-ridden pauses into powerful catalysts for a vibrant and fulfilling active aging journey. Remember, rest is not weakness, it's wisdom. Embrace it, and watch your body and spirit blossom with renewed energy and a newfound appreciation for the joy of movement, at any age.

Modifying Exercises: Cater to Your Body's Needs and Limitations

Modifying Exercises: Cater to Your Body's Needs and Limitations - A Dance of Strength and Grace

As we embark on the exhilarating journey of active aging, embracing challenges and pushing our boundaries becomes a daily mantra. Yet, in this quest for fitness, it's crucial to remember that our bodies, like well-loved books, whisper stories of their own. Each page holds tales of past experiences, whispers of strengths, and gentle reminders of limitations. It's in listening to these stories that we unlock the true magic of exercise: the art of modification.

Modifying exercises isn't a sign of weakness; it's a dance of strength and grace, a celebration of individuality, and a testament to the wisdom gained through years of living. It's about customizing your fitness routine to cater to your unique needs, ensuring that movement brings joy, not pain, and fuels sustainable progress, not frustration.

Understanding Your Body's Landscape:

Before embarking on the creative journey of modification, it's vital to map the landscape of your own body. This self-exploration involves:

- Identifying Strengths and Weaknesses: We all have areas where we shine and places where we're a bit more "under construction." Knowing your personal strengths, like exceptional flexibility or cardiovascular endurance, can help you leverage them in your workouts. Similarly, acknowledging limitations, like joint pain or reduced balance, allows you to choose exercises that bypass those hurdles without compromising your fitness goals.

- Listening to Pain Cues: Pain is a beacon, not a roadblock. If an exercise triggers sharp pain, listen to your body's plea for a shift. This doesn't mean abandoning the activity; it signifies the need for modification to make it safe and effective.

- Considering Medical Conditions: Some medical conditions necessitate specific modifications to avoid complications. Consult your doctor or a physiotherapist for personalized guidance and ensure your workout aligns with your medical needs.

The Art of Modification: A Toolbox of Options:

Now, with a map in hand, it's time to explore the vibrant toolbox of modification options. Remember, creativity is your key:

- Intensity Reduction: Dial down the intensity of an exercise without losing its essence. For example, swap high-impact jumps for controlled squats or opt for lighter weights in strength training.

- Range of Motion Adjustments: Modify the full range of motion of an exercise to suit your capabilities. Instead of deep lunges, try shallower steps or perform chair-supported squats.

- Equipment Alternatives: Use equipment strategically to provide support and stability. Replace push-ups with wall push-ups for less strain on your shoulders, or utilize resistance bands instead of free weights for controlled muscle engagement.

- Posture and Alignment: Proper posture and alignment are key to preventing injuries and maximizing benefits. If maintaining perfect form in a specific exercise feels tricky, modify it with adjustments that ensure your body stays safe and aligned.

- Breaking Down Movements: Complex exercises can be broken down into simpler components. Instead of full burpees, try separate squats, lunges, and push-ups for a gentler challenge.

- Focus on Form Over Formality: Perfection is a fleeting visitor, especially in the realm of exercise. Don't be afraid to adjust the form of an exercise to suit your needs. What matters most is safe and effective movement, not adhering rigidly to textbook examples.

Remember, Your Journey is Unique:

There's no one-size-fits-all approach to modification. Experiment, explore, and listen to your body. What works for your friend might not be your perfect fit, and that's okay. Embrace the individuality of your journey and celebrate the modifications that make exercise a source of joy, not a source of frustration.

Beyond the Physical:

Modification extends beyond just altering exercises. It encompasses a holistic approach to your well-being:

- Mindset Matters: Approach modification with a positive attitude. View it as an opportunity to discover new ways to move your body and celebrate your unique capabilities.

- Celebrate Progress: Don't compare your modified routine to someone else's unedited version. Track your own progress, acknowledge your improvements, and celebrate each step, big or small, on your personal fitness journey.

- Seek Support: Don't hesitate to seek guidance from a qualified fitness professional or physical therapist. They can provide personalized modifications and ensure you're on the right track.

Embrace the Dance of Modification:

Remember, active aging is not about pushing through limitations, but about dancing with them. Let the music of your body guide you, embrace the beauty of modifications, and discover the joy of movement that resonates with your unique rhythm. In this way, you'll cultivate a sustainable fitness practice that fuels your well-being, celebrates your individuality, and keeps you dancing gracefully through the years of vibrant life that lie ahead.

Bonus Tips for Modification Masters:

- Keep a modification journal: Document your modifications for each exercise, creating a personalized library of movements that work for you. This can be a valuable resource for future workouts and a source of inspiration for others.

- Turn modification into a game: Make it fun! Challenge yourself to come up with creative ways to modify exercises, using household items or your environment as props. This adds a playful element to your routine and keeps you engaged.

- Share your journey: Inspire others by sharing your successful modifications with friends, family, or online communities. You might just help someone else discover the beauty of movement that caters to their own unique needs.

- Embrace technology: Apps and online resources can offer a wealth of modified exercise options. Explore fitness platforms specifically designed for older adults or those with specific limitations to find inspiration and guidance.

- Never stop learning: As your body changes and your fitness goals evolve, so should your modifications. Stay open to new ideas, learn from others, and continue to refine your personal dance with movement throughout your active aging journey.

By incorporating these tips and embracing the spirit of modification, you can transform your fitness routine into a vibrant tapestry of personalized movement, one that celebrates your strength, respects your limitations, and fuels a lifelong pursuit of well-being. Remember, modification is not a weakness, it's a superpower. Own it, unleash its potential, and dance your way to a healthier, happier you, every step of the way.

Food Sensitivities and Dietary Restrictions: Making Healthy Choices for You

Food Sensitivities and Dietary Restrictions: Making Healthy Choices for You

In the vibrant tapestry of active aging, navigating the world of food can feel like deciphering an ancient code. Terms like "gluten-free," "lactose-intolerant," and "plant-based" swirl around us, leaving some wondering: "Where do I even begin?" But fear not, fellow adventurers! Your journey towards delicious and nourishing meals, tailored to your unique needs, is closer than you think. This chapter equips you with the knowledge and confidence to navigate the sometimes-murky waters of food sensitivities and dietary restrictions, ensuring your path to wellness is paved with flavor and satisfaction.

Understanding the Landscape:

Food sensitivities and dietary restrictions are as diverse as the individual stories they hold. Some, like allergies to peanuts or shellfish, trigger immediate and sometimes life-threatening reactions. Others, like lactose intolerance or gluten sensitivity, manifest in less dramatic, but still impactful ways. Additionally, personal choices, such as vegetarianism or veganism, shape the way we approach food. No matter the reason, acknowledging your unique dietary needs is the first step towards unlocking a world of healthy and delicious possibilities.

Exploring the Spectrum:

Let's delve into the spectrum of food sensitivities and dietary restrictions:

- Food Allergies: These triggers an immune response, inducing symptoms like hives, wheezing, or even anaphylaxis. Common allergens include peanuts, shellfish, milk, eggs, soy, wheat, and tree nuts. Identifying and completely avoiding your trigger foods is crucial for maintaining optimal health.

- Food Intolerances: Unlike allergies, intolerances don't involve the immune system. They occur when your body has difficulty digesting certain foods, like lactose in milk or gluten in wheat. Symptoms can range from digestive discomfort to fatigue and headaches. Finding alternative food sources or ways to manage digestion is key.

- Medical Conditions: Certain medical conditions may necessitate specific dietary modifications. For example, someone with diabetes might need to limit sugar intake, while another with high cholesterol might benefit from reducing saturated fat. Working with a healthcare professional ensures your diet aligns with your medical needs.

- Lifestyle Choices: Vegetarianism and veganism are dietary choices based on ethical and ecological considerations. Vegetarians abstain from meat, while vegans exclude all animal products, including dairy and eggs. Understanding the nutritional requirements of these choices helps ensure you get the essential nutrients your body needs.

The Art of Adaptation:

Adapting your diet doesn't have to feel like a daunting climb. Here are some tips for smooth sailing:

- Seek Guidance: Consult a registered dietitian or nutritionist to personalize your dietary plan and address any nutritional deficiencies.

- Embrace Variety: Explore alternative food sources within your dietary restrictions. For example, try almond milk instead of cow's milk or lentil pasta instead of wheat pasta.

- Label Reading 101: Become a master label decoder! Look for hidden triggers and opt for products clearly labeled according to your needs.

- Get Creative in the Kitchen: Experiment with recipes and discover exciting flavor combinations that fit your restrictions. You might be surprised at the delicious possibilities!

- Make it Social: Don't let your dietary needs isolate you. Share your journey with friends and family, and inspire them to explore healthy and delicious options together.

Remember, You're in Charge:

Making healthy choices for you doesn't mean sacrificing flavor or fun. Embrace your dietary needs as an opportunity to explore new taste horizons and celebrate your individuality. With knowledge, creativity, and support, you can navigate the world of food with confidence, paving your path to a vibrant and delicious journey of active aging.

Bonus Tips for Dietary Detectives:

- Keep a Food Journal: Track your meals and any associated symptoms to identify potential triggers and patterns.

- Plan Your Meals: Planning your meals in advance helps you make informed choices and avoid impulsive decisions.

- Stay Informed: Research upcoming food trends and new products on the market that might cater to your specific needs.

- Join Online Communities: Connect with others who share your dietary restrictions for support, advice, and recipe inspiration.

- Celebrate Small Wins: Focus on your progress, not perfection. Every healthy choice, no matter how small, is a step towards a more vibrant you.

Remember, navigating food sensitivities and dietary restrictions is a continuous journey of exploration and discovery. Embrace the adventure, celebrate your uniqueness, and above all, savor the delicious and nourishing possibilities that await!

Celebrating Progress, Not Perfection: Focus on Small Wins and Long-Term Goals

Celebrating Progress, Not Perfection: Focus on Small Wins and Long-Term Goals - A Symphony of Self-Appreciation

In the grand concert hall of active aging, the melody of progress can sometimes get drowned out by the insistent drumming of "shoulds" and "musts." We chase ever-elusive ideals, obsessing over the next milestone, the next pound shed, the next push-up conquered. And in this relentless pursuit of perfection, the joy of movement, the quiet whispers of our bodies, and the sweet melody of small victories often fade into the background. But it's time to change the tune, fellow adventurers! This chapter invites you to turn down the volume on self-criticism and crank up the joyous chorus of celebrating progress, not perfection.

Embracing the Imperfect Journey:

Let's face it, the path to optimal health is rarely a straight line. It's a winding road, paved with stumbles, setbacks, and triumphs both big and small. Perfection is a myth, a mirage shimmering under the relentless sun of comparison. The true magic lies in appreciating the imperfections, the detours, and the unexpected pit stops that shape our unique journeys. It's in the dance of progress, not the final pose, that we discover the true joy of active aging.

The Power of Small Wins:

In the quest for grand achievements, we often overlook the whispers of small victories. But it's these seemingly insignificant steps that lay the foundation for sustainable progress. Celebrating a completed walk instead of obsessing over marathon goals, savoring a healthy meal instead of lamenting a missed workout, acknowledging the quiet strength gained from climbing stairs instead of yearning for sculpted biceps – these are the cornerstones of a journey fueled by self-appreciation and sustainable change.

Redefining Success:

Shift your perspective. Success in active aging isn't about replicating magazine covers or conquering impossible challenges. It's about listening to your body, respecting its limitations, and celebrating every step you take towards a healthier, happier you. It's about the quiet satisfaction of moving your body in a way that feels good, the deliciousness of a nourishing meal shared with loved ones, the newfound energy that allows you to climb a hill without gasping for breath. These are the true trophies of your journey, the gold medals of self-care and mindful movement.

Tools for Celebrating:

Here are some ways to make self-appreciation the soundtrack of your journey:

- Acknowledge Your Wins: Keep a "progress journal" to track not just goals achieved, but also small victories like increased energy, improved mood, or simply showing up for your body.

- Reward Yourself: Celebrate milestones, big and small, with non-food rewards like a relaxing bath, a walk in nature, or spending time with loved ones.

- Visualize Success: Create a vision board depicting your long-term goals and small wins along the way. This serves as a constant reminder of your journey and the triumphs you've achieved.

- Practice Gratitude: Shift your focus from what you "should" be doing to what you are already doing. Be thankful for your body's strength, resilience, and capacity for movement.

- Embrace Imperfection: Celebrate the stumbles and setbacks as valuable lessons on your path. See them as opportunities to learn, adjust, and grow.

The Long-Term Symphony:

By focusing on small wins and celebrating progress, not perfection, you orchestrate a long-term symphony of self-appreciation and sustainable change. It's a melody that transcends fleeting achievements and resonates with the deep satisfaction of living a life in tune with your body and your values. So, turn down the volume on self-criticism, raise the curtain on your unique strengths, and dance to the joyous rhythm of progress, one small win at a time. Remember, perfection is a fantasy, but progress is a beautiful, empowering reality, and its music is waiting to be celebrated.

Bonus Tips for Progress Applause:

- Share your journey: Find a supportive community or friend to celebrate your wins with. Sharing your triumphs amplifies the joy and keeps you motivated.

- Focus on the process: Savor the experience of movement, the taste of nourishing food, the connection with your body. This takes the focus off the outcome and makes the journey itself rewarding.

- Challenge negative thoughts: Replace self-criticism with positive affirmations. Remind yourself of your progress, your strengths, and your commitment to well-being.

- Be kind to yourself: Treat yourself with the same compassion and encouragement you would offer a friend on their own journey.

- Remember, it's a marathon, not a sprint: Embrace the long-term perspective. Savor the small wins, learn from the stumbles, and keep moving forward, one mindful step at a time.

By incorporating these tips, you can transform your pursuit of health from a relentless quest into a joyful symphony of self-appreciation. You'll discover that the true treasure doesn't lie in reaching some imaginary finish line, but in the beautiful melodies of progress played out in every mindful movement, every healthy choice, and every small victory celebrated along the way. So, let the music of your journey begin, fellow adventurers! The stage is yours, and the spotlight awaits. Go forth, celebrate your progress, and dance to the vibrant rhythm of a life well-lived, one imperfect, magnificent step at a time.

Part 4: Bonus Chapters - Living Your Best Life After 60

Chapter 13: Sleep for Recovery and Well-Being: The Power of a Good Night's Rest

Creating a Relaxing Bedtime Routine: Winding Down for Quality Sleep

Creating a Relaxing Bedtime Routine: Winding Down for Quality Sleep - A Lullaby for Your Body and Mind

As the sun dips below the horizon, casting long shadows across our days, our bodies yearn for a different kind of light – the soft, soothing glow of a well-established bedtime routine. This nightly ritual, far from a mundane chore, is a powerful tool in the arsenal of active aging. It's a lullaby for our senses, a gentle guide leading us from the frenetic pace of the day to the restorative embrace of sleep, the cornerstone of well-being and vibrant living.

Why a Bedtime Routine Matters More After 60:

As we age, sleep patterns naturally shift. We may find ourselves falling asleep earlier and waking earlier, experiencing lighter or shorter sleep cycles. This is why a consistent bedtime routine becomes even more crucial. It helps regulate our internal clock, known as the circadian rhythm, promoting deeper, more restorative sleep and leaving us feeling energized and refreshed in the morning.

The Pillars of a Relaxing Routine:
Crafting your ideal bedtime routine is an act of self-discovery, a personalized symphony of calming activities that lull you towards sleep. Here are some key pillars to consider:

1. Setting the Stage:

- Dim the Lights: Gradually dim the lights in your bedroom as evening approaches. Opt for warm, soft light sources like lamps or candles instead of harsh overhead lighting.
- Tidy Up: A cluttered space can clutter your mind. Dedicate a few minutes to tidying your bedroom, creating a calm and soothing environment conducive to sleep.
- Embrace the Senses: Spritz calming scents like lavender or chamomile, play soothing music, or light aromatherapy candles to engage your senses and signal relaxation.
-

2. Winding Down the Mind:
- Disconnect and Unwind: Put away your screens at least an hour before bedtime. The blue light emitted by electronics suppresses melatonin production, the hormone that helps regulate sleep. Choose calming activities like reading a book, taking a warm bath, or journaling to quiet your mind.
- Practice Relaxation Techniques: Deep breathing exercises, meditation, or progressive muscle relaxation can help calm your nervous system and prepare your body for sleep.
- Limit Stimulating Activities: Avoid watching intense TV shows or engaging in heated debates before bed. Opt for soothing activities that promote tranquility and prepare your mind for slumber.
-

3. Nourishing Your Body:
- Eat a Light Dinner: Avoid heavy meals close to bedtime. Opt for a light, healthy dinner at least two hours before sleep to avoid indigestion and promote restful sleep.

- Stay Hydrated: Drink plenty of water throughout the day, but avoid large quantities close to bedtime to prevent frequent bathroom breaks.
- Avoid Stimulants: Limit caffeine and alcohol intake, especially in the evening. These substances can disrupt your sleep cycle and make it harder to fall asleep and stay asleep.
-

4. Establishing Consistency:

- Set a Regular Sleep Schedule: Go to bed and wake up at the same time each day, even on weekends. This helps regulate your circadian rhythm and promotes better sleep quality.
- Create a Sleep Ritual: Develop a consistent bedtime routine that includes calming activities like reading, taking a bath, or listening to music. This signals to your body that it's time to wind down and prepare for sleep.
- Make it a Priority: Treat your bedtime routine with the same respect as any other important appointment. Prioritize it in your schedule and avoid compromising on it unless absolutely necessary.
-

Bonus Tips for Sleep Symphony Conductors:

- Invest in a Comfortable Bed: Ensure your mattress and pillows provide adequate support and comfort. Consider using blackout curtains to block out any light that might disturb your sleep.
- Exercise Regularly: Physical activity can improve sleep quality, but avoid strenuous workouts close to bedtime. Opt for gentle exercise like yoga or walking in the evening.
- Seek Professional Help: If you experience persistent sleep problems, consult your doctor or a sleep specialist. They can

help identify any underlying medical conditions or recommend personalized sleep strategies.

•

Note: Remember, everyone's ideal bedtime routine is unique. Experiment with different activities and find what works best for you. Be patient and allow your body to adjust to the new routine.

Unknown Facts:

- Studies have shown that lavender oil can promote relaxation and improve sleep quality.
- Regular meditation can help reduce stress and anxiety, which can disrupt sleep.
- Taking a warm bath before bed can help lower your body temperature, making it easier to fall asleep.

Remember, a good night's sleep isn't a luxury, it's a necessity. By crafting a relaxing bedtime routine and making it a priority, you can unlock the power of sleep, fuel your well-being, and embrace the vibrant energy that active aging has to offer. So, dim the lights, quiet your mind, and let the lullaby of your routine guide you into the peaceful embrace of sleep. In the morning, you'll awake refreshed, revitalized, and ready to conquer the day with the renewed vigour that only a truly restorative night can bring. Remember, sleep is not a passive surrender to darkness, but an active investment in your health and happiness. Make it a cornerstone of your active aging journey, and watch your life blossom with energy, joy, and boundless possibilities.

Sweet dreams, fellow adventurers!

Addressing Sleep Challenges: Common Issues and Effective Solutions

Addressing Sleep Challenges: Common Issues and Effective Solutions - Restoring Harmony to Your Sleep Symphony

The symphony of a good night's sleep, crafted with a calming bedtime routine, can sometimes be disrupted by discordant notes: tossing and turning, persistent thoughts, or the unwelcome melodies of snoring. These sleep challenges, while frustrating, are common in all age groups, especially after 60. But fear not, fellow adventurers! Just like any complex musical composition, understanding the cause of the dissonance empowers you to find the right tune for restoring harmony to your sleep.

Common Sleep Disruptors:
Let's identify some of the most common sleep challenges faced by those over 60:

- Insomnia: Difficulty falling asleep or staying asleep can be caused by stress, anxiety, medical conditions, medications, or environmental factors.
- Early Morning Waking: Waking up too early and being unable to fall back asleep can be due to aging changes in sleep patterns, light exposure, or medical conditions.
- Sleep Apnea: This condition causes pauses in breathing during sleep, leading to fragmented sleep and daytime fatigue.

- Restless Legs Syndrome: An uncontrollable urge to move your legs, especially at night, can disrupt sleep and cause discomfort.
- Hot Flashes: These sudden surges of heat, common in menopause, can cause sweating and difficulty sleeping.

Finding the Right Note:

Now, let's explore some effective solutions for these sleep challenges:

- Insomnia:
  - Cognitive Behavioral Therapy (CBT) for Insomnia: This evidence-based therapy can help identify and change negative sleep thoughts and behaviors.
  - Relaxation Techniques: Deep breathing exercises, meditation, and progressive muscle relaxation can promote calmness and prepare your body for sleep.
  - Regular Exercise: Physical activity can improve sleep quality, but avoid strenuous workouts close to bedtime.
- Early Morning Waking:
  - Exposure to Bright Light: Get plenty of exposure to natural light during the day, especially in the morning.
  - Avoid Napping: Long or late-afternoon naps can make it harder to fall asleep at night.
  - Relaxing Wake-Up Routine: Avoid checking screens or jumping into busy tasks upon waking. Start your day with calming activities like light stretching or gentle yoga.
- Sleep Apnea:

- - Consult a Doctor: Early diagnosis and treatment of sleep apnea is crucial for improving sleep quality and reducing health risks.
  - CPAP Therapy: This common treatment uses a mask to deliver continuous positive airway pressure during sleep, keeping airways open.
  - Lifestyle Changes: Weight loss, avoiding alcohol and caffeine before bed, and sleeping on your side can help manage sleep apnea symptoms.
- Restless Legs Syndrome:
  - Warm Baths or Massages: These can help relax muscles and reduce the urge to move your legs.
  - Iron Supplements: Consult your doctor to determine if iron deficiency is contributing to your symptoms and consider appropriate supplementation.
  - Mind-Body Techniques: Yoga, meditation, and gentle stretching can help manage the discomfort and improve sleep quality.
- Hot Flashes:
  - Maintain a Cool Bedroom Temperature: Lower room temperature and use breathable bedding to alleviate overheating during the night.
  - Dress in Layers: Wear layers of clothing you can easily remove if you get hot during the night.
  - Limit Stimulants: Avoid caffeine and alcohol, which can worsen hot flashes and disrupt sleep.

Bonus Tips for the Sleep Orchestra:

- Seek Professional Help: Don't hesitate to consult a doctor or sleep specialist if your sleep problems persist or significantly impact your well-being.
- Keep a Sleep Diary: Track your sleep patterns, including bedtime, wake time, mood, and any activities that might be affecting your sleep. This can help identify potential triggers and inform treatment decisions.
- Celebrate Small Victories: Even small improvements in sleep quality can be beneficial. Be kind to yourself and celebrate your progress, no matter how gradual.

Note: Remember, individual experiences are unique. Consult your doctor to determine the best course of action for your specific sleep challenges.

Unknown Facts:

- Studies have shown that laughter can improve sleep quality. A good laugh before bed can help reduce stress and promote relaxation.
- Listening to calming music before bed can also be helpful for falling asleep. Choose soothing melodies or nature sounds to quiet your mind.
- Experiencing vivid dreams is more common in older adults and can be a normal part of the aging process. However, if your dreams are disruptive or disturbing, consult your doctor.

Remember, addressing sleep challenges is a journey, not a destination. Be patient, experiment with different solutions, and celebrate every step towards a more restful night. By restoring harmony to your sleep symphony, you'll unlock a vibrant chorus of well-being, energy, and renewed joy in the morning. So, tune out the discordant notes, embrace the lullaby of effective solutions, and prepare to dance to the rhythmic melody of a rejuvenated you. Sweet dreams, fellow adventurers, and may your sleep be as deep and harmonious as the music of your own well-being!

The Link Between Sleep and Exercise: How One Supports the Other

The Link Between Sleep and Exercise: How One Supports the Other - A Dance of Renewal in Every Step

Imagine two celestial bodies orbiting each other, their gravitational pull creating a harmonious cosmic dance. In the realm of well-being, sleep and exercise play a similar role, their intertwined rhythms fueling a vibrant melody of health and vitality. In this chapter, we embark on a journey of discovery, exploring the profound link between these two pillars of active aging, and how understanding their synergy empowers us to orchestrate a symphony of renewed energy and well-being in every step we take.
A Shared Language of Restoration:

Both sleep and exercise are potent tools for recovery and renewal. During sleep, our bodies and minds repair, replenish, and consolidate memories. Exercise, on the other hand, stimulates muscle growth, boosts metabolism, and enhances cognitive function. But the magic lies in their interconnectedness. Exercise enhances sleep quality, and adequate sleep fuels the energy and motivation for consistent movement. They become partners in a virtuous cycle, each amplifying the benefits of the other.

Exercise: The Lullaby for Your Nervous System:
Physical activity, even in gentle forms, can act as a natural lullaby for your nervous system. It promotes the release of calming hormones like serotonin and endorphins, reducing stress and anxiety

that can disrupt sleep. Regular exercise also helps regulate your circadian rhythm, the internal clock that governs your sleep-wake cycle, making it easier to fall asleep and stay asleep at night.

Sleep: The Fuel for Movement:
Think of sleep as the metabolic bank account for your body and mind. When you're well-rested, your energy levels are high, your muscles are primed for action, and your cognitive function is sharp. This translates to better performance in your workouts, improved endurance, and enhanced motivation to keep moving. Conversely, inadequate sleep depletes your energy reserves, making it harder to exercise and impacting your overall fitness goals.

The Benefits of Harmony:
The synergistic dance between sleep and exercise unlocks a wealth of benefits for active aging:

- Enhanced Mood and Mental Well-being: Both sleep and exercise combat stress and anxiety, leading to improved mood, better cognitive function, and a sharper memory.
- Increased Physical Fitness: When well-rested, you have the energy and stamina for more efficient workouts, leading to improved muscle strength, cardiovascular health, and overall fitness.
- Weight Management: Getting enough sleep helps regulate hormones that control appetite and metabolism, making it easier to maintain a healthy weight and boost your energy levels.
- Reduced Risk of Chronic Diseases: Adequate sleep and regular exercise work together to lower the risk of chronic conditions like heart disease, diabetes, and certain cancers.

- Stronger Immune System: Both sleep and exercise boost your immune system, making you more resistant to infection and illness, crucial for maintaining good health in your later years.

Creating a Balanced Symphony:

So, how do we orchestrate this beautiful dance between sleep and exercise? Here are some tips:

- Schedule your workouts strategically: Avoid strenuous exercise close to bedtime, as it can energize your body and make it harder to fall asleep. Opt for gentle activities like yoga or light stretching in the evening.
- Prioritize sleep hygiene: Maintain a consistent sleep schedule, create a relaxing bedtime routine, and ensure your bedroom is dark, quiet, and cool.
- Listen to your body: Adapt your exercise routine to your energy levels and sleep quality. If you're feeling tired, prioritize rest and adjust your workout intensity accordingly.
- Embrace the outdoors: Spending time in nature, especially during daylight hours, can help regulate your circadian rhythm and improve sleep quality.
- Seek professional guidance: If you have trouble sleeping or struggle to find the right balance between exercise and rest, consult your doctor or a sleep specialist.

Bonus Tip: Track your sleep and exercise patterns in a journal. This can help you identify correlations between your activity levels and sleep quality, allowing you to fine-tune your routine for optimal results.

Note: Remember, there's no one-size-fits-all approach to the sleep-exercise dance. Experiment, find what works best for you, and celebrate your progress. Every step you take towards a harmonious balance is a step towards a healthier, happier you.

Unknown Facts:
- Studies have shown that regular exercise can help older adults fall asleep faster and sleep more soundly.
- Even small amounts of physical activity, like taking short walks throughout the day, can significantly improve sleep quality.
- People who get enough sleep tend to be more active and exercise more regularly than those who are sleep-deprived.

Remember, sleep and exercise are not rivals, but teammates in the game of well-being. By understanding their interconnectedness and fostering their harmonious dance, you unlock a vibrant symphony of health, energy, and renewed vitality in every step you take. So, put on your dancing shoes, fellow adventurers, and let the rhythm of movement and the lullaby of a good night's sleep guide you on a journey of active aging filled with boundless possibilities. Embrace the power of this dynamic duo, and watch your life blossom with the joyous melody of renewed health, vibrant energy, and the exhilarating satisfaction of a life well-lived.

Sweet dreams and happy steps, adventurers! May your journey be paved with the harmony of sleep and exercise, leading you to a future brimming with well-being and the timeless beauty of an active, empowered you.

Getting Enough Rest: Prioritizing Sleep for Overall Health and Happiness

Getting Enough Rest: Prioritizing Sleep for Overall Health and Happiness - A Symphony of Self-Care

In the grand concert hall of active aging, where the melody of movement and the rhythm of laughter fill the air, there's a hidden instrument, crucial yet often overlooked: sleep. Its soft lullaby, while seemingly unassuming, plays a vital role in the harmonious symphony of overall health and happiness. This chapter invites you to step into the backstage of your own well-being, exploring the profound consequences of getting enough rest and unraveling the secrets to prioritizing sleep for a vibrant, joyful life.

The Orchestra of Health:

Imagine your body as a complex orchestra, where every organ and system plays a vital role in the symphony of well-being. When you deprive yourself of sleep, it's like silencing a key instrument, throwing the entire composition into disarray. Sleep isn't simply a passive time-out; it's a period of intense activity behind the scenes, where your body repairs, recharges, and prepares for the next act.

The Melody of Physical Rejuvenation:

During sleep, our bodies focus on cellular repair and tissue regeneration. Growth hormone production peaks, muscles rebuild from the wear and tear of daily activities, and the immune system ramps up its defenses. This nocturnal orchestra ensures you wake up feeling refreshed, strong, and ready to tackle the day with vigor.

Without adequate sleep, this vital repair work remains incomplete, leaving you feeling drained, achy, and vulnerable to illness.

The Rhythm of Mental Well-being:
Sleep plays a crucial role in managing stress, regulating emotions, and consolidating memories. It's like a mental spa, washing away the anxieties of the day and sharpening your cognitive functions. When sleep-deprived, our stress hormones surge, our emotions become volatile, and our thinking turns foggy. This disrupts our ability to concentrate, make decisions, and navigate the complexities of life.

The Harmony of Happiness:
The link between sleep and happiness is undeniable. Getting enough rest not only boosts your mood but also enhances your ability to savor life's pleasures. It fuels your creativity, sparks your humor, and gives you the energy to connect with loved ones and engage in activities that bring you joy. Conversely, chronic sleep deprivation can lead to irritability, depression, and a diminished sense of well-being, muffling the vibrant melody of happiness within you.

Prioritizing the Lullaby:
In a world that often glorifies busyness and sacrifices sleep for productivity, prioritizing rest can feel like a radical act. Yet, it's a revolution worth taking. Here are some harmonious tools to help you prioritize sleep:

- Establish a regular sleep schedule: Go to bed and wake up at the same time each day, even on weekends. This helps regulate your body's internal clock and makes it easier to fall asleep and wake up feeling refreshed.

- Create a relaxing bedtime routine: Wind down in the hour before bed with calming activities like reading, taking a warm bath, or listening to soothing music. Avoid screens and intense conversations, as they can stimulate your mind and make it harder to fall asleep.
- Optimize your sleep environment: Make sure your bedroom is dark, quiet, cool, and clutter-free. Invest in comfortable bedding and consider using blackout curtains if necessary.
- Exercise regularly: Physical activity can improve sleep quality, but avoid strenuous workouts close to bedtime, as they can energize your body and make it harder to fall asleep.
- Limit stimulants: Avoid caffeine and alcohol, especially in the evening, as they can disrupt your sleep patterns.
- Seek professional help: If you experience persistent sleep problems, consult your doctor or a sleep specialist. They can help identify any underlying medical conditions or recommend personalized sleep strategies.

Bonus Tip: Keep a sleep diary to track your sleep patterns, habits, and any factors that might be affecting your sleep. This can help you identify triggers and adjust your routine accordingly.

Note: Remember, the optimal amount of sleep varies from person to person. Most adults need between 7-9 hours of sleep per night to function optimally. Pay attention to your body's cues and adjust your sleep schedule accordingly.

Unknown Facts:
- Studies have shown that sleep deprivation can impair your driving skills as much as alcohol intoxication.

- Regular sleep can boost your creativity and problem-solving abilities.
- Laughter before bed can actually improve sleep quality by reducing stress and promoting relaxation.

Remember, sleep is not a luxury, it's a necessity. By prioritizing rest and making it a cornerstone of your daily routine, you invest in your physical, mental, and emotional well-being. You invite the lullaby of sleep to join the symphony of your life, amplifying the melodies of health, happiness, and the boundless joy of active aging. So, silence the noise of busyness, tune in to your body's rhythms, and let the powerful song of sufficient sleep guide you towards a vibrant future where every day dawns as a fresh composition, filled with the exhilarating notes of well-being and the resounding chorus of a life well-lived. Sweet dreams, fellow adventurers, and may your journey be serenaded by the gentle lullaby of rest, leading you ever closer to the harmonious masterpiece of active aging.

Chapter 14: Stress Management for Inner Peace: Tools for a Calm and Balanced Mind

Recognizing Stressors: Identifying What Triggers Your Response

Recognizing Stressors: Identifying What Triggers Your Response

Stress, that unwelcome companion, can creep into our lives in a thousand different ways. It can lurk in deadlines, arguments, traffic jams, or even seemingly insignificant worries. But before we can tackle this unwelcome guest, we must first identify its calling card: recognizing our stressors, those specific situations or thoughts that trigger our stress response. This chapter is your guide to becoming a detective of your own inner landscape, uncovering the hidden agents that set your stress alarm blaring.

Unmasking the Culprits:

1. Physical Sensations: Our bodies often speak louder than words. Listen for the telltale signs of stress: a clenched jaw, a racing heart, sweaty palms, or tight shoulders. These physical manifestations can be early warnings, alerting you to potential stressors before they overwhelm you.

2. Emotional Shifts: Notice sudden changes in your mood. Do you become irritable, restless, or anxious in certain situations? Does a specific topic trigger feelings of guilt, anger, or despair? Identifying these emotional patterns can pinpoint hidden stressors impacting your well-being.

3. Behavioral Changes: Observe if your behavior changes under stress. Do you withdraw from social interaction, resort to unhealthy coping mechanisms like overeating or excessive screen time, or become prone to procrastination? These actions could be subconscious attempts to escape your stressors, signaling the need for a closer look.

Digging Deeper:

Beyond physical, emotional, and behavioral cues, delve deeper into the inner dialogue that fuels your stress. Ask yourself:

- What thoughts or situations precede my stress response? Is it the looming deadline, the upcoming family gathering, or the unresolved conflict with a colleague? Identifying the specific triggers helps you understand the source of your stress.

- What are the underlying beliefs fueling my stress? Do you hold unrealistic expectations of yourself or others? Do you catastrophize? Uncovering these hidden beliefs can provide opportunities for reframing and positive self-talk.

- Are there recurring themes in my stressors? Do money worries, interpersonal conflicts, or health concerns consistently trigger your stress response? Recognizing these patterns can reveal areas in your life that need greater attention or a proactive approach.

Bonus Tip: Keep a stress journal! Track your physical sensations, emotions, and thoughts alongside the situations that provoke them. Over time, patterns will emerge, helping you identify your unique stress triggers.

Note: Not all stressors are external. Internal factors like negative self-talk, perfectionism, and chronic worry can also trigger our stress response. Pay attention to your inner critic and learn to challenge its unproductive whispers.

Unknown Fact: Laughter is a powerful antidote to stress! Find activities that bring you genuine joy and laughter, whether it's spending time with loved ones, watching a funny movie, or pursuing a hobby.

Remember: Identifying your stressors is the first crucial step towards managing them effectively. By becoming a keen observer of your body, mind, and emotions, you gain the power to disarm those hidden triggers and cultivate a calmer, more balanced state of mind.

The journey to inner peace begins with self-awareness. Explore, identify, and disarm your stressors, and step into a life less burdened by the unwelcome guest of stress.

In the next section, we'll delve into practical tools and techniques to effectively manage your stress response. Stay tuned!

Relaxation Techniques: Deep Breathing, Meditation, Mindfulness Exercises

Relaxation Techniques: Deep Breathing, Meditation, and Mindfulness Exercises

We've identified the culprits, those pesky stressors lurking in our lives. Now, it's time to equip ourselves with the antidote: a potent arsenal of relaxation techniques designed to quell the stress response and cultivate inner peace. In this chapter, we'll explore three powerful tools:

1. Deep Breathing: Your On-Demand Tranquility Tool

Imagine this: a simple breath in, a gentle breath out, and with each cycle, the tension melts away, replaced by a wave of calm. That's the magic of deep breathing, a readily available stress-buster you can wield anytime, anywhere.

Why it works: Deep breathing activates the parasympathetic nervous system, our body's "rest and digest" mode. This counteracts the stress-induced fight-or-flight response, lowering heart rate, blood pressure, and cortisol levels.

How to do it: Find a quiet place, sit comfortably with your back straight, and close your eyes if you wish. Slowly inhale through your nose for a count of 4, feeling your belly expand. Hold for a count of 2, then exhale slowly through pursed lips for a count of 6. Repeat for 5-10 minutes, focusing on the rhythm of your breath and letting go of distracting thoughts.

Bonus Tip: Try visualizing your breath as calming blue light entering your body with each inhale, and radiating golden warmth as you exhale. This adds a layer of mental imagery to enhance the relaxation effect.

Unknown Fact: Studies show that deep breathing can be as effective as medication in reducing anxiety and depression symptoms. So, take a deep breath, you powerful being!

2. Meditation: Cultivating Inner Silence

Imagine a still lake reflecting the moonlight, undisturbed by ripples. That's the essence of meditation: training your mind to find stillness amidst the constant chatter of thoughts and emotions.

Why it works: Meditation activates the prefrontal cortex, the brain's control center, enhancing focus, clarity, and emotional regulation. It also strengthens the connections between brain regions responsible for learning, memory, and empathy, fostering greater well-being.

How to do it: There are many meditation styles, but a simple beginner's practice is mindfulness meditation. Sit comfortably, close your eyes (optional), and focus on your breath without judgment. When your mind wanders, gently bring your attention back to your breath. Start with short sessions of 5-10 minutes and gradually increase as you become more comfortable.

Note: Don't get discouraged if your mind feels like a runaway train at first! Observe your thoughts without judgment, like watching clouds pass by the sky. With practice, you'll find moments of stillness and peace within the storm.

Bonus Tip: Try guided meditations for beginners. Many apps and online resources offer recordings that gently guide you through the process, making it easier to learn and maintain the practice.

3. Mindfulness Exercises: Anchoring Yourself in the Present

Mindfulness is like bringing a spotlight to the present moment, paying attention to your thoughts, emotions, and sensations without judgment. This simple act can be a powerful tool for managing stress and anxiety.

Why it works: Mindfulness breaks the cycle of rumination and worry, grounding us in the present where there are no deadlines, conflicts, or worries – just the breath, the sounds around you, the feel of your clothes on your skin. This shift in perspective offers immediate relief from stress.

How to do it: Start with simple mindfulness exercises. Take a mindful walk, focusing on the sensations of your feet touching the ground, the breeze on your skin, and the sounds of nature. Or, savor a mindful meal, paying attention to the colors, textures, and flavors of each bite. You can also practice mindful stretching or gentle yoga, combining movement with awareness.

Unknown Fact: Mindfulness improves cognitive flexibility, meaning you become better at adapting to change and managing stress effectively. It's like building an inner resilience muscle.

Bonus Tip: Download a mindfulness app with short exercises you can integrate into your daily routine, like mindful breathing while waiting in line or a brief body scan before going to sleep.

Remember: Relaxation techniques are not magic bullets, but powerful tools in your stress-management arsenal. Experiment with different methods, find what resonates with you, and incorporate them into your daily life. With consistent practice, you'll cultivate a greater sense of inner peace and resilience, empowering you to navigate life's inevitable stressors with grace and ease.

In the next section, we'll explore additional tools and strategies for building your stress-management toolkit. Stay tuned!

Staying Connected: Social Interaction and Support Systems for Reduced Stress

Staying Connected: Social Interaction and Support Systems for Reduced Stress

We may strive for individual strength and resilience, but the truth is, humans are wired for connection. In the face of stress, our deepest need is not to face it alone. This chapter explores the potent antidote of social interaction and support systems in bolstering our well-being and mitigating the grip of stress.

Why Connecting Matters:

- Oxytocin, the "love hormone": Social interaction triggers the release of oxytocin, a neurotransmitter that promotes feelings of calmness, trust, and empathy. This natural high helps buffer the stress response and fosters emotional resilience.

- Shared burdens, lighter shoulders: Talking about your burdens with a trusted friend or family member can lighten the load. Supportive connections provide an outlet for emotions, offering valuable perspective and reducing the feeling of being overwhelmed.

- Belonging and validation: Feeling part of a supportive community provides a sense of belonging and validation. Knowing you're not alone in your struggles fosters confidence and encourages seeking help when needed.

Building Your Support Network:

- Nurture existing relationships: Invest time and energy in deepening connections with loved ones. Share your concerns, offer support in return, and relish moments of laughter and joy together.

- Embrace the power of "tribe": Seek out communities that share your interests or hobbies. Join a book club, a fitness class, or online forums. Engaging with like-minded individuals creates a sense of belonging and fosters new, supportive connections.

- Don't underestimate professional help: Consider seeking therapy or joining a support group for stress management. Therapists can provide tools and strategies for coping with stress, while support groups offer a safe space to share experiences and receive validation from peers.

Beyond Talk: Embracing Different Forms of Connection:

- Physical touch: A warm hug, holding hands, or even a pat on the back can release oxytocin and offer nonverbal reassurance. Engage in these forms of touch with loved ones to experience its stress-reducing power.

- Acts of kindness: Offering help to others is a powerful way to connect and foster a sense of purpose. Volunteer in your community, perform random acts of kindness, or simply be there for someone in need. These acts not only benefit the recipient but also lower your own stress levels.

- Nature as a healer: Immerse yourself in the beauty of nature. Take a walk in the park, hike in the woods, or simply sit by a peaceful pond. Connecting with nature offers a sense of awe and can significantly reduce stress and anxiety.

Bonus Tip: Prioritize quality time over quantity. Deep, meaningful conversations with a few close confidantes can be more beneficial than attending crowded social gatherings. Choose connections that resonate with you and nourish your soul.

Note: Building a strong support network takes time and effort. Be patient with yourself and embrace the journey of connection. Remember, even small interactions can have a significant impact on your well-being.

Unknown Fact: Studies show that social isolation is a major risk factor for stress, anxiety, and even physical health problems. So, reach out, connect, and experience the transformative power of human connection in mitigating stress and cultivating inner peace.

Staying connected offers a powerful shield against the onslaught of stress. By nurturing existing relationships, seeking new connections, and embracing various forms of social interaction, we weave a safety net of support that empowers us to navigate life's challenges with greater resilience and joy. Remember, you are not alone, and within your community lies a wealth of support waiting to be embraced.

Saying No: Setting Boundaries and Prioritizing Yourself

Saying No: Setting Boundaries and Prioritizing Yourself

In the face of an overflowing schedule, demanding requests, and endless to-do lists, the word "no" can feel like a forbidden utterance. Yet, within this simple negation lies a powerful tool for stress management and cultivating inner peace: the art of setting boundaries and prioritizing yourself. This chapter delves into the liberating act of saying no, empowering you to reclaim your time, energy, and well-being.

Why Saying No Matters:

- Combating Overload: Our stress response thrives on feeling overwhelmed. Saying no allows you to manage your commitments, preventing your plate from piling high with unrealistic expectations.

- Protecting Your Resources: Time, energy, and mental bandwidth are precious. Saying no to unnecessary demands ensures you have adequate resources to invest in activities that truly matter to you and nourish your well-being.

- Honoring Your Values: When you say yes to everything, you say no to your own wants and needs. Setting boundaries aligns your commitments with your values, ensuring your life reflects what truly matters to you.

- Boosting Self-Esteem: Saying no can feel scary, but it's an act of self-care and self-respect. Setting boundaries reinforces your worth and prioritizes your well-being, sending a powerful message to yourself and others.

Saying No with Grace and Clarity:

- Be honest and direct: Clearly explain why you're declining, whether it's lack of time, conflicting commitments, or simply needing to prioritize yourself. Be respectful but firm in your message.

- Offer alternatives: If appropriate, suggest an alternative solution or timeframe for revisiting the request. This demonstrates your willingness to help while maintaining your boundaries.

- Practice saying no without justifications: You don't always need to explain yourself! A simple, polite "no, thank you" is perfectly sufficient. Remember, your time and energy are valuable, and you don't need to apologize for prioritizing them.

Bonus Tip: Practice saying no in low-pressure situations. Start by declining invitations you're less enthusiastic about, building your confidence and comfort with expressing your limits.

Note: Saying no can be challenging, especially if you struggle with people-pleasing tendencies or fear of disappointing others. Remember, setting boundaries is not about being selfish; it's about being responsible for your well-being and creating a sustainable, fulfilling life.

Unknown Fact: Studies show that people who effectively set boundaries experience lower levels of stress, anxiety, and burnout. Saying no is an investment in your mental and physical health!

Embrace the "Yes" that Follows:

Saying no paves the way for saying yes to what truly matters. Prioritizing your well-being and setting boundaries empowers you to invest your time and energy in activities that bring you joy, nourish your soul, and contribute to your overall well-being. This "yes" is the cornerstone of a fulfilling life, a life fueled by purpose and personal satisfaction.

Saying no is not a rejection, it's a redirection. It's a powerful declaration of self-care and an act of liberation that empowers you to navigate life with greater purpose, ease, and inner peace. Remember, you have the right to prioritize yourself, and by setting boundaries, you pave the way for a life brimming with the "yeses" that truly matter.

Chapter 15: The Joy of Movement: Embracing Activities You Love

Dancing: Express Yourself and Get Your Heart Rate Up

For many people, the word "dance" conjures images of graceful ballerinas or electrifying hip-hop routines. But the truth is, dancing is for everyone, regardless of age, skill level, or physical limitations. And for those over 60, embracing the joy of movement through dance can be a transformative experience, offering a wealth of benefits for both body and mind.

Dancing for Physical Fitness:

- Cardio Boost: Dancing gets your heart rate up, improving cardiovascular health and endurance. Whether you're swaying to a slow ballad or busting a move to a lively salsa tune, your body is getting a workout. Regular dancing can lower blood pressure, reduce the risk of heart disease, and increase energy levels.

- Strength and Flexibility: Different dance styles engage different muscle groups. Ballroom dancing strengthens your core and improves balance, while Latin dance tones your legs and hips. Even gentle swaying can improve flexibility and range of motion, reducing the risk of falls and injuries.

- Bone Health: Dancing, particularly weight-bearing styles like tap or line dancing, helps build and maintain bone density, which is crucial for preventing osteoporosis as we age.

Dancing for Mental Well-being:

- Stress Relief: Putting on your favorite music and letting loose on the dance floor is a fantastic way to relieve stress and tension. Dancing releases endorphins, the body's natural feel-good chemicals, leaving you feeling happy and uplifted.

- Mind-Body Connection: Dancing requires focus and coordination, engaging both your physical and mental faculties. This can improve cognitive function, memory, and overall brain health. The repetitive nature of some dance styles can also be meditative, calming the mind and promoting relaxation.

- Social Connection: Dancing is often a social activity, providing opportunities to connect with others, make new friends, and combat loneliness. Joining a dance class or simply dancing with your partner can bring joy and laughter into your life and strengthen your social bonds.

Finding Your Groove:

There's a dance style out there for everyone, so don't be afraid to experiment and find what makes you move. Here are some suggestions for those over 60:

- Ballroom dancing: Waltz, foxtrot, and swing are elegant and sophisticated choices that offer excellent cardiovascular and core strengthening benefits.

- Latin dance: Salsa, merengue, and bachata are lively and fun, with infectious rhythms that get your heart pumping and your hips shaking.

- Line dancing: A great option for solo dancers or social groups, line dancing is easy to learn and offers a low-impact workout that improves coordination and balance.

- Zumba: Combining Latin dance rhythms with fitness moves, Zumba is a high-energy, calorie-burning workout that's perfect for those who want to get their groove on with a group.

Bonus Tips:

- Start slow and listen to your body: Don't push yourself too hard, especially if you're new to dancing. Begin with shorter sessions and gradually increase the intensity and duration as your fitness improves.

- Wear comfortable shoes and clothing: Choose supportive shoes with good cushioning and clothing that allows freedom of movement.

- Make it fun!: Don't take yourself too seriously. Laugh, smile, and enjoy the music and the movement. Dancing should be a joyful experience, not a chore.

- Find a supportive community: Join a dance class, meetup group, or online forum for older adults who love to dance. Having others around you who share your passion can be motivating and inspiring.

Note: If you have any health concerns, consult your doctor before starting any new exercise program, including dancing.

Unknown Facts:

- Studies have shown that dancing can improve cognitive function in people with Alzheimer's disease and dementia.

- Dancing can also help reduce the risk of depression and anxiety, promoting overall mental well-being.

- The oldest competitive ballroom dancer in the world is Fay Compton, who is 93 years old!

So, put on your dancing shoes, turn up the music, and let loose! Embrace the joy of movement and discover the many benefits that dancing can bring to your life, both physically and mentally. You might just surprise yourself with the hidden dancer within you!

Gardening: Connecting with Nature and Enjoying Physical Activity

For those seeking both physical activity and a deep connection with nature, gardening offers a treasure trove of benefits. It's more than just digging in the dirt and watching things grow; it's a symphony of movement, mindfulness, and sensory delight for the mind, body, and soul.

A Gentle Workout Disguised as Play:

Unlike rigorous gym routines, gardening is a gentle, low-impact activity that engages your entire body in subtle yet effective ways. Here's how you reap the fitness rewards:

- Bending and squatting: Planting seeds, weeding, and harvesting involve constant bending and squatting, strengthening your core muscles, improving flexibility, and boosting balance.

- Cardio boost: Pushing a wheelbarrow, carrying seedlings, and walking around your plot work wonders for your heart rate and cardiovascular health.

- Upper body workout: Digging, pruning, and raking engage your arms, shoulders, and back, building strength and improving agility.

- Vitamin D boost: Spending time outdoors soaking up the sunshine helps your body synthesize essential Vitamin D, crucial for bone health and boosting mood.

Beyond the Physical: A Feast for the Senses:

Gardening offers a multi-sensory experience that transcends mere exercise. Let your senses get pampered:

- Sight: Witnessing the vibrant colours of blooming flowers, the lush greenery of thriving leaves, and the delicate beauty of butterflies fluttering by is a feast for the eyes.

- Smell: Breathe in the intoxicating fragrance of freshly turned earth, blooming roses, and ripe herbs – a natural aromatherapy session that soothes the soul.

- Touch: Feel the cool earth beneath your fingers, the smooth texture of ripe tomatoes, and the gentle prickle of leaves – a grounding experience that connects you to nature.

- Sound: Listen to the chirping of birds, the buzzing of bees, and the rustling of leaves in the wind – a symphony of nature that calms the mind and inspires peace.

Mindfulness on a Green Canvas:

Gardening transcends physical movement; it's a practice in mindfulness. Focusing on the present moment, tending to your plants, and nurturing life fosters a sense of calm and reduces stress. The repetitive nature of certain tasks becomes meditative, allowing your mind to wander while your hands work diligently.

A Social Playground for Green Thumbs:

Gardening doesn't have to be a solitary act. Invite friends and family to join you for a planting party, share your harvest, or swap gardening tips. Social interaction not only adds to the fun but also motivates you to stay active and engaged.

Tips for Gardening Success:

- Start small and gradually increase your activity level.

- Listen to your body and take breaks when needed.

- Use ergonomic tools that minimize strain and fatigue.

- Choose tasks that align with your fitness level and interests.

- Make it fun! Play music, listen to podcasts, or sing along to the birds.

Bonus Tips:

- Plant low-maintenance flowers and vegetables to minimize heavy lifting.

- Build raised garden beds to reduce bending and kneeling.

- Use a gardening stool or kneel on a padded mat for comfort.

- Invest in comfortable shoes and clothing that allow for freedom of movement.

Note: If you have any pre-existing health conditions, consult your doctor before starting any new physical activity program, including gardening.

Unknown Facts:

- Studies have shown that gardening can significantly reduce stress hormones like cortisol and boost mood-enhancing endorphins.

- Spending time in nature, like gardening, can improve cognitive function and memory.

- Regular gardening can decrease the risk of developing chronic diseases like heart disease, diabetes, and some cancers.

So, grab your gloves, dig your fork into the soil, and let the joy of gardening bloom. Embrace the gentle movement, the sensory delights, and the mindful connection with nature. Your body, mind, and spirit will thank you for it. Happy gardening!

Hiking and Exploring: Outdoor Adventures for Body and Mind

For those seeking an invigorating blend of physical activity, breathtaking scenery, and mental stimulation, lacing up your boots and hitting the trail offers a treasure trove of benefits. Hiking and exploration are not just about conquering peaks or reaching the next waypoint; they are a tapestry woven with movement, mindfulness, and connection to the natural world, enriching both body and mind.

A Physical Playground for All Ages:

Hiking caters to a wide range of fitness levels, making it an accessible and adaptable activity for those over 60. Whether you choose gentle nature walks or challenging mountain climbs, the benefits are undeniable:

- Cardio boost: Ascending slopes and navigating terrain elevates your heart rate, improving cardiovascular health and endurance.

- Strength and balance: Uneven paths and inclines engage your core muscles, legs, and ankles, enhancing overall strength and balance.

- Bone health: Walking on different surfaces stimulates bone density, a crucial factor in preventing osteoporosis in later life.

- Vitamin D boost: Soaking up the sunshine while hiking helps your body synthesize essential Vitamin D, vital for bone health and mood regulation.

Mindfulness on the Move:

Beyond the physical, hiking offers a meditative escape from the daily grind. Immersing yourself in nature fosters mindfulness, reducing stress and anxiety. The rhythmic sound of your footsteps, the rustling leaves, and the chirping of birds create a natural soundtrack for introspection and relaxation.

Unleashing the Explorer Within:

Hiking invites you to be an adventurer, a cartographer of your own journey. Each trail presents a new challenge, a puzzle to solve, and a landscape to discover. The sense of accomplishment upon reaching a summit or finding a hidden waterfall is a powerful motivator and a reminder of your own inner strength and resilience.

Connecting with Nature's Symphony:

Hiking opens your senses to the wonders of the natural world. Breathtaking vistas, vibrant wildflowers, the earthy scent of the forest, and the gentle melody of a babbling brook – each element of nature awakens your senses and fosters a deep connection to the environment.

Tips for Enjoyable Hikes:

- Choose trails that match your fitness level and interests. Start with shorter, easier trails and gradually build up your endurance.

- Plan your hike thoroughly. Research the trail length, difficulty level, and weather conditions.

- Pack appropriately. Wear comfortable shoes and clothing with layers for changing weather. Bring plenty of water, sunscreen, and a first-aid kit.

- Go with a group or buddy. This adds safety and social interaction, making the hike more enjoyable.

- Leave no trace. Respect the environment by packing out all your trash and minimizing your impact on the trail.

Bonus Tips:

- Use trekking poles for stability and balance on uneven terrain.

- Take breaks when needed and enjoy the scenery.

- Pack healthy snacks and a light lunch to fuel your body for longer hikes.

- Capture the beauty of your journey with photos or journaling.

Note: If you have any pre-existing health conditions, consult your doctor before starting any new physical activity program, including hiking.

Unknown Facts:

- Studies have shown that spending time in nature can significantly reduce stress hormones like cortisol and boost mood-enhancing endorphins.

- Hiking can improve cognitive function and memory, especially in older adults.

- Regular outdoor activity can strengthen the immune system and reduce the risk of chronic diseases.

So, grab your backpack, lace up your boots, and step onto the path less traveled. Embrace the physical challenge, the mental clarity, and the profound connection with nature that hiking offers. Let the mountains guide you, the forests inspire you, and the journey itself become your reward. Happy trails!

Volunteering: Giving Back and Staying Active in Your Community

For those seeking an activity that combines physical movement with the profound satisfaction of giving back, volunteering offers a unique blend of benefits. It's more than just helping others; it's a potent cocktail of physical activity, social connection, and purpose, enriching both your body and your spirit.

Moving with a Mission:

Volunteering doesn't have to be confined to sedentary tasks. Many opportunities provide a surprising workout while making a difference. Consider these options:

- Habitat for Humanity: Build homes alongside others, engaging in carpentry, painting, and general construction tasks, providing a full-body workout for a worthy cause.

- Animal shelters: Walk dogs, clean kennels, and play with furry friends, getting your daily dose of cardio and animal therapy.

- Park clean-up: Pick up litter, rake leaves, and plant trees, enjoying the fresh air and sunshine while beautifying your community.

- Delivering meals: Ride bikes or walk routes to deliver meals to the elderly or homebound, combining errands with gentle exercise.

- Gardening at community projects: Dig, plant, and tend to community gardens, reaping the physical benefits of gardening while contributing to fresh, local produce.

Beyond the Body: Boosting Mind and Spirit:

Volunteering isn't just about burning calories. It offers a wealth of non-physical benefits:

- Social connection: Combatting loneliness and isolation, volunteering fosters interaction with like-minded individuals and strengthens community bonds.

- Purpose and meaning: Contributing to a cause bigger than yourself provides a sense of purpose and fulfillment, boosting self-esteem and overall well-being.

- Reduced stress: Helping others and being part of a supportive community can significantly reduce stress and anxiety, improving mental health.

- Cognitive stimulation: Learning new skills, planning projects, and interacting with diverse people can keep your mind sharp and engaged.

- Sense of accomplishment: Witnessing the impact of your work and celebrating milestones with others creates a powerful sense of achievement and motivation.

Tips for Finding Your Volunteer Niche:

- Identify your interests: What are you passionate about? Animal welfare, environmental causes, education? Find an organization that aligns with your values.

- Consider your physical limitations: Choose activities that match your fitness level and abilities. Start small and gradually increase your time and intensity.

- Be flexible: Don't be afraid to try different roles and organizations until you find the perfect fit.

- Connect with others: Join volunteer groups or teams to share experiences, find support, and make new friends.

- Have fun! Remember, volunteering should be enjoyable and rewarding. Embrace the positive vibes and let your good deeds fuel your journey.

Bonus Tip:

- Partner up with a friend or family member for volunteer activities. Enjoy mutual motivation, shared laughter, and strengthen your relationships while giving back.

Note:

- When choosing volunteer opportunities, ensure they prioritize the safety and well-being of all participants, including older adults.

Unknown Facts:

- Studies have shown that volunteering can significantly reduce the risk of depression and anxiety, especially in older adults.

- Engaging in regular volunteer activities can boost cognitive function and memory, potentially reducing the risk of dementia.

- The social connections forged through volunteering can strengthen the immune system and improve overall health.

So, step outside your comfort zone, lace up your walking shoes, and embrace the powerful combination of movement, community, and purpose that volunteering offers. You'll be surprised by the positive impact it has on your body, mind, and spirit, enriching your life and the lives of those around you. Remember, even small acts of kindness can make a big difference. Happy volunteering!

Chapter 16: Mental Fitness Matters: Keeping Your Brain Sharp and Engaged

Brain Training Games and Activities: Puzzles, Crosswords, Memory Challenges

Staying sharp and engaged as we age isn't just about physical activity; it's also about keeping our minds active and challenged. Just like our bodies, our brains benefit from regular exercise, and engaging in brain training activities can offer a plethora of benefits. Not only can it help improve memory, focus, and problem-solving skills, but it can also boost mood, enhance creativity, and even delay the onset of cognitive decline associated with aging.

One of the most accessible and enjoyable ways to keep your brain active is through brain training games and activities. These activities come in a variety of forms, from classic pen-and-paper puzzles to sophisticated online apps and games. Here are some popular options to explore:

1. Puzzles and Crosswords:

- Crosswords: These classic word puzzles challenge your vocabulary, memory, and logic skills. They come in varying difficulty levels, so you can find one that suits your current abilities and gradually increase the challenge as you improve.

- Sudoku: This number-placement puzzle requires concentration, logical deduction, and strategic thinking. Filling in the grids with the correct numbers while adhering to the rules provides a satisfying mental workout.

- Jigsaw Puzzles: Putting together a jigsaw puzzle is a relaxing and visually stimulating activity that exercises your spatial reasoning and problem-solving skills. Completing a large puzzle can be a rewarding accomplishment and a great conversation starter.

- Logic Puzzles: These puzzles present brainteasers and riddles that require critical thinking and creative problem-solving. They can be enjoyed alone or with a partner, making them a fun way to exercise your brain while socializing.

2. Memory Challenges:

- Memory Games: These games, like matching pairs or remembering sequences, test your short-term memory and visual recall. Many online platforms offer memory games with increasing difficulty levels and different themes, keeping things fresh and engaging.

- Learning a New Language: Embracing the challenge of learning a new language is a fantastic way to keep your brain sharp. It forces you to learn new vocabulary, grammar rules, and sentence structures, keeping your mind active and engaged.

- Memorizing Poems or Quotes: This traditional method of memory training remains effective. Choose poems or quotes that resonate with you and challenge yourself to memorize them. Reciting them regularly can strengthen your recall abilities and keep your mind active.

3. Online Brain Training Programs:

- Lumosity: This popular platform offers a variety of brain training games and exercises that target different cognitive skills. The program personalizes your training based on your performance, keeping things challenging and engaging.

- Elevate: This app combines brain training games with reading comprehension and critical thinking exercises. It provides insights into your cognitive strengths and weaknesses, allowing you to tailor your training program accordingly.

- Fit Brains: This program offers a diverse selection of brain training games, from memory challenges to logic puzzles and visual exercises. It provides different difficulty levels and tracks your progress, keeping you motivated to improve.

Bonus Tips:

- Mix it up: Don't stick to the same type of brain training activity all the time. Variety is key to keeping your brain engaged and challenged. Try different puzzles, games, and activities to work out different cognitive skills.

- Schedule regular sessions: Make brain training a part of your routine. Dedicate short periods each day, even if it's just 15-20 minutes, to engaging in brain training activities. Consistency is key to reaping the benefits in the long run.

- Have fun! Brain training shouldn't feel like a chore. Choose activities you find enjoyable and engaging. The more you enjoy the process, the more likely you are to stick with it and see results.

Note: While brain training games and activities offer numerous benefits, it's important to note that they are not a cure-all for cognitive decline. If you have concerns about your memory or cognitive function, it's always best to consult with a healthcare professional.

Unknown Facts:

- Studies have shown that engaging in brain training activities can lead to increased brain volume in areas associated with memory and executive function.

- Playing brain games can also improve brain connectivity, meaning the various parts of your brain communicate more effectively with each other.

- Even short bursts of brain training can have positive effects. A study found that just 15 minutes of brain training per day for three months led to improvements in memory and processing speed.

Remember, keeping your mind active and engaged is crucial for overall well-being as we age. By incorporating brain training games and activities into your routine, you can not only sharpen your cognitive skills but also enjoy the mental stimulation and sense of accomplishment they provide. So, grab a puzzle, open a brain training app, or challenge yourself to learn a new language – your brain will thank you for it!

Learning New Skills: Expand Your Horizons and Challenge Yourself

While brain training games and puzzles are fantastic tools, stepping outside the realm of dedicated cognitive exercises offers another powerful way to keep your mind sharp and engaged: embracing the challenge of learning new skills. This isn't just about memorizing facts; it's about pushing yourself beyond your comfort zone and opening doors to new possibilities.

Why is learning new skills beneficial for brain health?

- Neuroplasticity: Our brains are incredibly adaptable, capable of forming new neural connections throughout life. Learning new skills stimulates this process, creating fresh pathways and strengthening existing ones.

- Cognitive Flexibility: As you grapple with new concepts and procedures, your brain becomes more adept at adapting to different situations and solving problems creatively. This flexibility is crucial for maintaining mental agility as we age.

- Enhanced Memory: The process of learning new things strengthens memory formation and retrieval, helping you remember details and information more effectively.

- Sense of Accomplishment: Mastering a new skill brings immense satisfaction and a boost to self-confidence. This sense of achievement can motivate you to continue learning and keep your mind engaged.

So, what new skills can you explore? The possibilities are endless! Here are a few ideas to get you started:

- Pick up a new language: Learning a new language is not just about memorizing vocabulary and grammar; it's about understanding a different culture and perspective. It can be challenging, but the rewards are immense, from enhanced cognitive abilities to improved global communication skills.

- Take a musical instrument: Whether you've always dreamed of playing the piano or simply want to try your hand at the ukulele, learning an instrument is a fantastic way to exercise your brain, improve coordination, and boost your mood. The creative process of making music is also incredibly rewarding.

- Master a new technology: Don't be intimidated by the latest gadgets! Learning how to code, edit videos, or navigate social media platforms can be surprisingly engaging and intellectually stimulating. The skills you acquire can also open up new opportunities for work or hobbies.

- Embrace the art world: Painting, drawing, sculpting – the world of art offers endless possibilities for creative expression. Engaging in artistic pursuits can unleash your inner artist, stimulate your imagination, and improve hand-eye coordination.

- Become a culinary adventurer: Learning new cuisines or mastering advanced cooking techniques can be a delicious way to challenge your brain. It involves experimentation, problem-solving, and attention to detail, all while satisfying your taste buds.

- Dive into the world of writing: Whether you've always dreamed of writing your own novel or simply want to improve your communication skills, writing is a fantastic way to exercise your brain and express your creativity. Start a journal, write short stories, or join a writing group to share your work and receive feedback.

Bonus Tip: Don't be afraid to fail! Learning new skills involves making mistakes and overcoming challenges. Embrace the learning process, celebrate small victories, and remember that every misstep is an opportunity to grow and improve.

Note: Learning new skills doesn't have to be expensive or time-consuming. Many online resources offer free courses and tutorials, and local community centers often host affordable classes and workshops. The key is to find something that interests you and sparks your curiosity.

Unknown Facts:

- Studies have shown that learning a new language can delay the onset of dementia and Alzheimer's disease.

- Playing a musical instrument can improve memory, attention span, and even spatial reasoning skills.

- Learning new skills can help reduce stress and anxiety, contributing to overall mental well-being.

Remember, keeping your brain active and engaged is just as important as physical exercise for maintaining optimal health as we age. So, step outside your comfort zone, embrace the challenge of learning something new, and watch your mind blossom with newfound possibilities!

Social Interaction: Conversation, Games, and Staying Connected

While physical activity offers myriad benefits for our bodies and minds, human beings are inherently social creatures, and our well-being thrives on meaningful connections. In the context of movement, incorporating aspects of social interaction can not only enhance your enjoyment but also boost your mental and emotional well-being.

The Power of Social Interaction:

- Enhanced Motivation: Sharing your fitness journey with others, be it a workout buddy, a group exercise class, or even an online community, can provide a powerful source of motivation. The mutual encouragement, shared successes, and friendly competition can push you further and make exercise more enjoyable.

- Reduced Stress and Anxiety: Social interaction helps release endorphins, the body's natural feel-good chemicals, which combat stress and anxiety. Engaging in conversations, laughter, and playful banter during physical activities can significantly improve your mood and overall well-being.

- Cognitive Stimulation: Conversational exchanges, especially those involving problem-solving, humor, and storytelling, keep your brain active and engaged. Participating in games like charades, trivia, or even word games during group activities can further enhance cognitive function and memory.

- Combating Loneliness and Isolation: As we age, social connections become even more crucial for mental and emotional health. Regular interactions with friends, family, or like-minded individuals through activity-based gatherings can combat feelings of loneliness and isolation, contributing to a sense of belonging and community.

Ways to Integrate Social Interaction into Your Movement Routine:

- Join a group fitness class: Whether it's Zumba, yoga, swimming, or even dance classes, group activities provide a fantastic opportunity to exercise alongside others, build camaraderie, and share motivating energy.

- Create a workout buddy system: Find a friend or family member who shares your fitness goals and schedule regular workout sessions together. Having someone to exercise with can increase accountability, boost enjoyment, and add a playful competitive element.

- Organize sports or game nights: Gather friends and family for activities like badminton, volleyball, board games, or even charades. Combining physical activity with friendly competition and laughter is a fun and engaging way to socialize and stay active.

- Connect with online communities: Join online forums or groups dedicated to fitness for people over 60. Sharing tips, experiences, and motivating messages with like-minded individuals can provide a sense of support and connection even when exercising alone.

- Volunteer your time: Engaging in physical activities while giving back to the community is a fulfilling way to combine movement with meaningful social interaction. Volunteer at a local park for clean-up activities, participate in charity walks or runs, or offer your skills at an organization that needs them.

Bonus Tip: Don't be afraid to initiate! Stepping outside your comfort zone and introducing yourself to others in group settings can open doors to new friendships and expand your social circle. Be an active participant in conversations, share your own experiences, and be open to trying new activities.

Note: Social interaction doesn't have to be limited to in-person activities. Technology can also play a role in fostering connections. Video calls with friends or family members while engaging in individual exercises like walking or yoga can still provide a sense of connection and shared experience.

Unknown Facts:

- Studies have shown that social interaction can significantly improve cognitive function and memory, especially in older adults.

- Strong social connections are associated with a reduced risk of developing dementia and Alzheimer's disease.

- Loneliness and isolation have been linked to increased stress, anxiety, and depression, highlighting the importance of social interaction for overall well-being.

Remember, movement and social connection are essential ingredients for a happy and fulfilling life after 60. Embrace the joy of sharing your physical activities with others, cultivate meaningful connections, and watch your physical and mental health flourish!

Additional Resources:

- Meetup: https://www.meetup.com/: https://www.meetup.com/ (website for finding local groups and activities)

- Nextdoor: https://nextdoor.com/: https://nextdoor.com/ (platform for connecting with neighbors)

- Volunteering Match: https://www.volunteermatch.org/: https://www.volunteermatch.org/ (website for finding volunteer opportunities)

- AARP: https://www.aarp.org/: https://www.aarp.org/ (resources and information for people over 50)

So, step outside, join a group, strike up a conversation, and let the joy of movement and connection fuel your journey to a healthier and happier you!

Reading and Writing: Stimulate Your Mind and Express Yourself Creatively

Beyond puzzles and brain training games, two powerful tools for keeping your mind sharp and engaged are readily available: reading and writing. These seemingly simple activities offer a wealth of benefits for cognitive function, emotional well-being, and creative expression, making them invaluable pursuits for anyone seeking to maintain mental fitness after 60.

Why is reading beneficial for brain health?

- Enhanced Cognitive Function: Reading regularly stimulates various brain regions, improving memory, concentration, and critical thinking skills. The act of decoding words, following storylines, and understanding complex concepts strengthens neural pathways and keeps your mind agile.

- Vocabulary Expansion and Language Skills: Exposure to diverse written works enriches your vocabulary and strengthens your grasp of grammar and syntax. This not only improves communication skills but also enhances cognitive flexibility and problem-solving abilities.

- Reduced Stress and Anxiety: Immersing yourself in a captivating story can be a powerful tool for stress reduction. Reading provides an escape from daily worries, calms the mind, and triggers the release of endorphins, promoting feelings of relaxation and well-being.

- Improved Memory and Focus: Engaging with different narrative styles and information-dense texts strengthens your memory and concentration. The effort of comprehending complex plots, retaining details, and following arguments trains your brain to stay focused and process information efficiently.

Writing: Unleashing Creativity and Sharpening the Mind

While reading opens doors to new worlds and perspectives, writing allows you to create your own. Putting pen to paper (or fingers to keyboard) offers a unique set of benefits for mental fitness:

- Stimulates Creative Expression: Writing is an outlet for self-expression, allowing you to explore your thoughts, feelings, and imagination. Whether you pen a personal journal, craft stories, or engage in poetry, writing helps you tap into your creative potential and unlock new ways of thinking.

- Enhances Cognitive Flexibility: The process of writing involves brainstorming, organizing ideas, and formulating coherent sentences. This challenges your brain to be flexible, shift perspectives, and make connections between seemingly disparate concepts.

- Improves Communication Skills: Writing hones your ability to communicate effectively. You learn to articulate your thoughts clearly, choose the right words for your audience, and structure your ideas in a logical and engaging way.

- Boosts Memory and Cognitive Reserve: Regularly engaging in writing activities strengthens your memory and builds cognitive reserve, which protects your brain against age-related decline and neurodegenerative diseases.

Beyond the benefits:

Reading and writing offer several additional advantages for individuals over 60. Joining a book club can foster social interaction and combat loneliness. Writing memoirs or family histories can preserve precious memories and leave a legacy for future generations. Volunteering to write letters or stories for children or elders can add purpose and meaning to your life.

Bonus Tip: Don't be afraid to explore different genres and styles! Step outside your comfort zone and try reading historical fiction, biographies, or even poetry. Experiment with different forms of writing, from journaling and short stories to blogging and creative non-fiction.

Note: Reading and writing shouldn't feel like a chore. Choose materials that genuinely interest you and make the process enjoyable. Set realistic goals, start small, and celebrate your progress, no matter how incremental.

Unknown Facts:

- Studies have shown that reading regularly can slow down cognitive decline and reduce the risk of dementia and Alzheimer's disease.

- Writing, particularly expressive writing, can improve emotional well-being and reduce symptoms of depression and anxiety.

- Engaging in both reading and writing has been linked to a reduced risk of developing cognitive decline in older adults.

Remember, keeping your mind active and engaged is just as important as physical exercise for maintaining optimal health and well-being as we age. So, pick up a book, unleash your inner writer, and watch your mental fitness flourish!

Additional Resources:

- Your local library: A treasure trove of books and often hosts book clubs and author events.

- Online writing communities: Platforms like Medium or Wattpad offer opportunities to share your work and connect with other writers.

- Creative writing classes: Offered at community centers, senior centers, and online, these classes provide a supportive environment to hone your writing skills and meet like-minded individuals.

Open a book, grab a pen, and embark on a journey of intellectual and creative exploration. Your mind will thank you for it!

Chapter 17: Building a Support System: Finding Your Tribe and Sharing Your Journey

Joining Fitness Groups: Exercise and Socialization Combined

Staying motivated on your fitness journey after 60 isn't always a solo act. While personal commitment is crucial, finding a supportive network can make all the difference. One powerful way to do this is by joining a fitness group specifically designed for people over 60. These groups offer a unique blend of exercise and social interaction, creating a dynamic environment that can fuel your motivation, enhance your workouts, and even reshape your social life.

Benefits of Joining a Fitness Group:

- Enhanced motivation: Surrounding yourself with people of similar goals and challenges can create a contagious energy. Seeing others push themselves encourages you to do the same, fostering a sense of camaraderie and shared progress.

- Socialization and connection: Combatting loneliness and isolation is particularly important in later life. Fitness groups provide a welcoming space to connect with like-minded individuals, build friendships, and combat feelings of isolation. Sharing laughter, stories, and post-workout coffee boosts your mood and overall well-being.

- Variety and expertise: Group fitness classes often offer a diverse range of activities, from low-impact aerobics and strength training to dance and yoga. This exposes you to new workout styles, preventing boredom and keeping your routines fresh. Experienced instructors guide you through proper form and modifications, ensuring safety and maximizing results.

- Accountability and encouragement: Committing to regular group sessions adds an element of accountability, making it harder to skip workouts. The positive reinforcement and cheers from fellow group members keep you on track and celebrate your achievements, fostering a sense of belonging and community.

- Social support beyond the gym: The bonds forged in fitness groups often extend beyond the exercise class. Group outings, coffee dates, and even travel adventures can blossom, enriching your social life and creating lasting connections.

Finding the Right Fitness Group:

- Consider your interests and fitness level: Do you prefer gentle walks or more vigorous workouts? Are you drawn to dance, water aerobics, or strength training? Choose a group that aligns with your fitness preferences and physical limitations.

- Location and schedule: Look for groups that meet at convenient times and locations, fitting seamlessly into your daily routine.

- Trial classes and open days: Many groups offer introductory sessions or open days. Try out a few different options to find the one that resonates with you and where you feel comfortable.

- Ask around: Get recommendations from friends, family, or your local community center. Online forums and social media groups dedicated to fitness for over 60 can also be a valuable resource.

Making the Most of Your Fitness Group Experience:

- Introduce yourself and get to know others: Be open and friendly, actively participating in conversations and introductions. Don't be afraid to put yourself out there and build connections.

- Offer support and encouragement: Just as you appreciate receiving it, be an encouraging presence for others. Celebrate their successes and offer a helping hand when needed.

- Share your story and challenges: Vulnerability can be a powerful tool in building trust and deeper connections. Sharing your fitness goals and challenges allows others to relate and offer advice or support.

- Be open to trying new things: Don't be afraid to step outside your comfort zone and try new activities offered by the group. You might discover a hidden passion or a workout routine you never knew you'd enjoy.

- Organize social events: Take initiative and suggest group outings, potlucks, or other social activities outside the gym. This strengthens bonds and fosters a sense of community.

Bonus Tip: Consider volunteering for group events or taking on leadership roles within the group. This can boost your confidence, give back to the community, and deepen your connection with the members.

Note: Remember, not every group is a perfect fit. If you don't feel comfortable or welcome, don't hesitate to try another one. Finding the right group is key to maximizing your experience and reaping the full benefits of this valuable support system.

Unknown Fact: Studies have shown that social interaction and belonging are just as important for physical health as diet and exercise. Joining a fitness group can combat loneliness and isolation, reducing stress and boosting the immune system, further enhancing your overall well-being.

Joining a fitness group after 60 can be a transformative experience. It's more than just about exercise; it's about finding your tribe, building meaningful connections, and discovering a sense of belonging. So, lace up your walking shoes, put on your smile, and step into the exciting world of group fitness. You might just surprise yourself with the friendships, motivation, and joy you find along the way.

Finding a Workout Buddy: Motivation and Accountability

Finding Your Fitness Friend: Unleashing the Synergy of Sweat and Support

The road to fitness can be a winding path, filled with moments of inspiration and inevitable dips in motivation. We sweat, we struggle, and sometimes, we falter. But what if you didn't have to walk this path alone? What if alongside the burn of a challenging workout, you had the cheering embrace of a dedicated partner, a kindred spirit who shares your goals, celebrates your victories, and lifts you up on those days when the weights feel a little heavier, the treadmill a little longer? Enter the workout buddy, a dynamic force in your fitness journey, capable of transforming your solo struggle into a shared symphony of sweat, support, and unwavering motivation.

Why does a workout buddy hold the key to unlocking a winning fitness experience? Here's the breakdown:

- Double Dose of Motivation: One workout buddy equals two sets of lungs cheering you on, two pairs of high fives celebrating your triumphs. Their presence becomes a beacon of encouragement, pushing you beyond your comfort zone, and reminding you why you embarked on this journey in the first place. When the inner couch potato whispers sweet nothings about skipping that morning run, your buddy becomes the chorus of angels singing praises of accountability and shared accomplishment.

- Accountability Powerhouse: No more gym ghosting! A workout buddy adds a layer of friendly pressure, ensuring you show up and give it your all. Knowing someone is waiting for you at the gym, rain or shine, becomes a powerful deterrent against the siren song of procrastination. Accountability transcends the physical; it extends to sharing meal plans, discussing fitness goals, and offering healthy nudges when your diet choices threaten to stray from the path.

- Shared Struggles, Shared Triumphs: The journey to fitness is not always smooth sailing. There will be days when the burpees feel like torture, the miles stretch to an unending horizon. But with a workout buddy, you face these challenges together. Laughter mutes the burn, shared groans become a bonding experience, and celebrating milestones together amplifies the joy of achievement. Knowing you have someone who understands your struggles and shares your triumphs creates a powerful sense of camaraderie, making the journey feel less like a solo climb and more like a fun-filled hike with a friend.

- Beyond the Gym Walls: The magic of a workout buddy extends beyond the confines of the gym. From planning healthy social outings to sharing inspirational fitness articles, your workout buddy becomes an extension of your support system. They act as your fitness cheerleader, celebrating your non-gym victories, from conquering those extra flights of stairs to resisting the donut temptation at work. This holistic approach to well-being creates a positive ripple effect, enhancing your entire lifestyle and solidifying your commitment to a healthier you.

Crafting Your Winning Workout Buddy Duo:

- Seek Similar Souls: The key to a successful workout buddy partnership lies in compatibility. Look for someone with similar fitness goals, workout styles, and schedules. A running enthusiast paired with a yoga devotee might create scheduling clashes, while an introverted exerciser paired with a gym-loving extrovert might find their needs unmet.

- Communication is Key: Open and honest communication is vital. Discuss goals, workout preferences, and expectations upfront. Be there for each other, offering support and encouragement, but also respectfully understanding personal limitations and challenges. Honest feedback, delivered with kindness, can be invaluable for growth and progress.

- Celebrate Big and Small: Every milestone, from that extra half-mile on the treadmill to mastering a challenging yoga pose, deserves recognition. Celebrate each other's successes, acknowledging the hard work and dedication that goes into every victory. These shared celebrations not only strengthen your bond but also fuel your collective motivation to keep pushing forward.

- Respect Individuality: Remember, your workout buddy is not your carbon copy. Be mindful of their individual needs and preferences. Allow for differences in pace, workout styles, and even recovery times. Embrace your individuality while supporting each other on your unique paths to fitness.

Bonus Tip: Don't be afraid to step outside your comfort zone! Expand your search to fitness classes, online communities, or even neighborhood running groups. You might just find your perfect workout buddy where you least expect it.

Note: Not everyone clicks with someone on the first try. If your initial workout buddy partnership doesn't feel right, don't give up! Explore other options, and remember, finding the right person is half the victory.

Unknown Fact: Studies have shown that having a workout buddy can lead to increased exercise adherence, improved fitness outcomes, and even greater enjoyment of physical activity. So, what are you waiting for? Go out there, find your fitness friend, and unlock the synergy of sweat and support on your journey to a healthier, happier you!

Remember, your fitness journey is not a solo affair. Embrace the power of a workout buddy, and experience the transformative joy of shared motivation, unwavering accountability ...and a camaraderie that makes the path to well-being not just a struggle, but a shared adventure.

Together, you can laugh through lunges, high five through hurdles, and conquer every challenge with the knowledge that you have someone by your side, cheering you on every step of the way. So, let your workout buddy become your fitness confidante, your sweaty soulmate, your partner in progress. Because with a friend by your side, the road to fitness is not just about reaching your goals; it's about creating memories that will last a lifetime.

Beyond the Gym: Unleashing the Full Potential of Your Fitness Duo

While pushing each other at the gym is the foundation of your fitness friendship, the magic of your workout buddy extends far beyond the weight room walls. Here are some ways to unleash the full potential of your dynamic duo and take your wellness journey to the next level:

- Healthy Foodie Adventures: Embark on culinary explorations together, seeking out healthy cafes, trying new recipes, and whipping up nutritious meals in each other's kitchens. Support each other's healthy eating goals, offering tips, substituting ingredients, and motivating each other to ditch the junk food and embrace the wholesome goodness.

- Nature Escapes: Trade the treadmill for a trail, the elliptical for a scenic hike. Explore nature together, challenging yourselves with outdoor activities like kayaking, rock climbing, or even a simple walk in the park. Fresh air, stunning scenery, and shared physical exertion create a natural boost for your health and well-being, forging memories that go beyond the confines of the gym.

- Mind-Body Bliss: Partner up for yoga classes, meditation sessions, or even deep breathing exercises. Discover the power of connecting with your inner selves together, reducing stress, and finding balance in your fast-paced lives. These mind-body practices complement your physical training, creating a holistic approach to well-being and strengthening your bond on a deeper level.

- Motivational Meltdown Party: Feeling drained? Have a dedicated "motivation meltdown party" where you vent your frustrations, share your fitness struggles, and offer each other supportive words and laughs. Sometimes, all it takes is a good dose of understanding and a dash of humor to reignite your inner fire and get back on track.

- Celebrating Milestones (Big and Small): From conquering that challenging workout to finally mastering that headstand, every milestone deserves a celebration. Treat yourselves to healthy meals, organize a fun activity, or simply raise a glass (of water, of course!) to your achievements. These shared celebrations fuel your motivation, solidify your bond, and make your fitness journey a delightful one.

Remember, your workout buddy is your partner in this journey, not a competitor. Embrace their strengths, support their weaknesses, and together, create a synergy that propels you both towards a healthier, happier you. So, lace up your sneakers, grab your water bottles, and step out into the world, knowing that your fitness friend is right there beside you, every step of the way. You've got this, together!

Online Communities: Connecting with Like-Minded People Over 60

Beyond the Screen: Unveiling the Joy of Connection in Online Communities for the Over-60 Crowd

For decades, society has painted a bleak picture of aging – loneliness, isolation, and disconnection from the vibrant pulse of life. But for the remarkable generation over 60, defying stereotypes and embracing newfound freedoms, technology is bridging the gap, opening doors to a world of connection and camaraderie through online communities. Forget bingo nights and senior centers (though they have their charm!). Today, tech-savvy seniors are logging on, tapping away on keyboards, and discovering the electrifying world of virtual tribes where age is not a barrier, but a badge of honor.

Why are online communities a secret weapon for well-being and joy for the over-60 crowd? Here's the breakdown:

- Breaking the Loneliness Barrier: No more isolated evenings or quiet weekends. Online communities offer a gateway to a bustling world of like-minded individuals, ready to share, connect, and support. From lively forums buzzing with conversations to intimate chat groups focused on specific interests, there's a virtual space for everyone, where loneliness fades and a sense of belonging flourishes.

- Discovering Shared Passions: Whether you're an avid painter yearning for critique, a seasoned traveler itching to swap stories, or a budding baker seeking recipe inspiration, online communities cater to every passion imaginable. Find your tribe of amateur astronomers discussing constellations, join a virtual book club dissecting historical novels, or connect with fellow gardening enthusiasts sharing tips and blooming triumphs. This shared space rekindles your passions, ignites curiosity, and keeps your mind and spirit young.

- Embracing Lifelong Learning: Never stop learning! Online communities provide a platform for continuous intellectual stimulation and skill development. Join online courses on everything from coding to creative writing, participate in webinars about health and wellness, or engage in lively discussions about current affairs. These communities keep your mind sharp, expand your horizons, and prove that the pursuit of knowledge knows no age limit.

- Combating Technophobia: Forget the outdated image of seniors struggling with smartphones. This generation is embracing technology with gusto! Online communities provide a safe space to learn new skills, overcome tech hurdles, and connect with a tech-savvy support network. From navigating social media platforms to mastering video conferencing tools, the over-60 crowd is proving that age is just a number when it comes to embracing the digital world.

- Building Global Connections: The world shrinks and boundaries dissolve in the interconnected tapestry of online communities. Forge friendships with fellow seniors across continents, sharing cultural experiences, exchanging recipes from across the globe, and celebrating each other's triumphs no matter the distance. These virtual connections broaden your perspective, break down cultural barriers, and remind you that the human spirit of connection transcends borders and limitations.

Navigating the Labyrinth of Online Communities:

- Find Your Niche: With countless online communities vying for your attention, finding the right fit is crucial. Explore platforms like Reddit, Facebook groups, or dedicated websites catered to specific interests. Look for communities with an active user base, positive and respectful communication, and a shared passion for your chosen topic.

- Embrace the Learning Curve: Don't be intimidated by technology! Take online tutorials, seek help from younger family members, or join beginner-friendly forums. Remember, every tech guru was once a novice, and the journey of learning can be just as rewarding as the destination.

- Mind Your Safety: As with any online space, caution is key. Never share personal information, be wary of scams, and report any suspicious activity to the moderators. Remember, trust your instincts and prioritize your safety above all else.

- Be an Active Participant: Don't be a wallflower! Share your thoughts, experiences, and expertise. Ask questions, engage in discussions, and offer support to fellow members. Your active participation strengthens the community and enriches the experience for everyone.

- Embrace Real-Life Connections: Online communities are not meant to replace real-life interactions. Use them as a springboard to connect with like-minded individuals offline. Organize local meetups, participate in community events, or simply invite your virtual friends for coffee. Let the online spark ignite lasting friendships in the real world.

Bonus Tip: Not all communities are created equal. Don't hesitate to leave a community that feels negative, disrespectful, or unwelcoming. There are countless others waiting to embrace you with open arms.

Note: Remember, online communities are just one facet of a fulfilling life. Maintain a healthy balance between virtual connections and real-life interactions, hobbies, and personal pursuits.

Unknown Fact: Studies have shown that online social engagement can improve mental well-being, cognitive function, and overall health outcomes in older adults. So, don't be afraid to dive into the world of online communities! You might just discover a vibrant, supportive tribe waiting to welcome you with open hearts and shared passions.

Embrace the digital wave, over-60 adventurers! Step out of the shadows of societal stereotypes and into the sunlit realm of online communities. Here, laughter echoes across virtual borders, friendships bloom across screens, and minds dance to the rhythm of shared passions. No longer confined by physical limitations, you are citizens of a global village, where age is not a barrier, but a shared badge of wisdom and experience.

Beyond the Forums: Unleashing the Full Potential of Your Virtual Tribe

While lively forums and chat groups ignite the initial spark of connection, the magic of online communities unfolds in a tapestry of possibilities that extend far beyond the screen. Here are some ways to unleash the full potential of your virtual tribe and weave a richer, more vibrant experience:

- Virtual Travel Adventures: Embark on journeys around the world, armchair-style! Join online groups dedicated to virtual tourism, sharing travel photos, exchanging stories about favorite destinations, and planning future adventures together. From scaling the Himalayas online to exploring the Great Barrier Reef from your living room, your virtual tribe becomes your passport to a boundless world.

- Mastermind Groups for Growth: Tap into the collective wisdom and experience of your like-minded peers. Form small, focused groups based on shared goals, whether it's mastering a new skill, launching a creative project, or simply navigating the challenges of aging. Offer each other guidance, support, and constructive criticism, creating a space for mutual growth and shared triumphs.

- Creative Collaborations Unleashed: Let your artistic sparks fly in the digital crucible! Join online writing groups, share your artistic creations in dedicated forums, or even collaborate on virtual music projects. The supportive environment of your online community fosters creativity, pushes you beyond your comfort zone, and opens doors to unexpected artistic collaborations.

- Live Events that Bridge the Virtual Gap: Take your online friendships offline! Organize local meetups, plan group outings, or even host virtual events like online book readings or cooking demonstrations. These real-life connections add a tangible dimension to your virtual bonds, solidifying friendships and creating lasting memories.

- Mentorship and Reverse Mentorship: Age is not a one-way street! Share your life wisdom and expertise with younger members of your community, acting as mentors in areas like navigating family relationships, building successful careers, or simply appreciating the finer things in life. Conversely, embrace the tech-savviness and fresh perspectives of younger members, learning new skills and staying connected to the evolving digital landscape.

Remember, your online community is not just a collection of usernames; it's a living, breathing ecosystem. Be an active participant, offer your unique perspective, and contribute to the collective well-being of your virtual tribe. Celebrate diversity, embrace differences, and foster a space where respect, kindness, and open communication reign supreme.

So, log on, adventurers of the over-60 generation! The tapestry of online communities awaits your vibrant threads. Weave your stories, share your passions, and let your laughter echo across the digital landscape. In this world of boundless connections, remember, you are not alone. You are part of a vibrant tribe, united by the spirit of adventure, the joy of learning, and the unwavering belief that the best chapter of life is yet to be written. Go forth, connect, and embrace the boundless possibilities that lie beyond the screen!

Sharing Your Story: Inspiring Others and Finding Encouragement

Finding Your Voice, Sharing Your Light: The Transformative Power of Sharing Your Story

We all possess within us a unique tapestry of experiences, woven with threads of joy and sorrow, triumph and vulnerability. These stories, deeply personal and often unspoken, hold the power to resonate, to inspire, and to connect us on a level that transcends differences. Yet, so many of us keep these narratives tucked away, buried beneath layers of self-doubt or fear of judgment. What if, however, sharing your story could not only enrich the lives of others but also become a source of unexpected strength and connection for yourself?

Why does sharing your story hold the key to unlocking a powerful and transformative experience? Here's the illumination:

- Connecting in Vulnerability: When we share our struggles, failures, and moments of doubt, we chip away at the walls of isolation. Others recognize their own vulnerabilities reflected in our words, fostering empathy, understanding, and a sense of shared humanity. In this vulnerability, we forge profound connections, dismantling the illusion of separateness and reminding ourselves that we are not alone in our journey.

- Inspiring Courage: Our stories, both triumphant and challenging, have the power to ignite a spark of hope in others. By sharing our personal journeys of overcoming obstacles, achieving goals, or simply navigating life's twists and turns, we inspire courage in those who face similar challenges. Our voice becomes a beacon of possibility, whispering, "If I can do it, so can you."

- Finding Unexpected Healing: The act of sharing your story can be a powerful form of self-healing. As we articulate our experiences, we gain a new perspective, identifying patterns, processing emotions, and even finding humor in the midst of hardship. By giving voice to our inner struggles, we begin to understand them, integrate them into our narrative, and ultimately move beyond them with a renewed sense of self-compassion.

- Empowering Authenticity: Sharing our stories, in all their messy, unfiltered glory, is an act of radical self-acceptance. We embrace our flaws, celebrate our quirks, and own our experiences, flaws and all. This vulnerability paves the way for others to do the same, creating a ripple effect of authenticity and reminding us that it is in our imperfections that we find true connection and belonging.

- Building Stronger Communities: When we share our stories, we contribute to a richer tapestry of human experience. Our unique narratives become threads woven into the fabric of our communities, creating a kaleidoscope of perspectives, challenges, and triumphs. This collective wisdom not only strengthens our social bonds but also fosters understanding, tolerance, and a sense of shared purpose.

Crafting Your Path to Story-Sharing:

- Find Your Safe Space: Not everyone feels comfortable baring their soul to the world. Start small, sharing your story with close friends, family members, or even a trusted therapist. As you gain confidence, consider online communities dedicated to specific struggles or personal growth, where anonymous sharing can be a stepping stone to wider visibility.

- Embrace Imperfection: Don't strive for polished prose or a perfectly curated tale. Real stories are raw, messy, and sometimes even humorous. Focus on authenticity, on capturing the essence of your experience, not on crafting a literary masterpiece. Remember, your vulnerability is your strength.

- Find Your Purpose: What message do you want to convey? Is it a story of resilience, of hope, or simply a window into a unique perspective? Identifying your purpose helps you tailor your sharing and ensures your message resonates with those who need it most.

- Seek Support and Feedback: Sharing your story can be an emotional journey. Lean on your support network, seek feedback from trusted individuals, and remember that constructive criticism is an opportunity for growth, not judgment. The right kind of support can embolden your voice and refine your message.

- Embrace the Ripple Effect: Never underestimate the power of your story. Even the smallest ripple can reach far and wide, impacting lives you may never know. Share your story with confidence, knowing that your voice has the potential to inspire, heal, and connect in ways you could never imagine.

Bonus Tip: Remember, storytelling is a continuous journey. As you evolve and grow, your story evolves with you. Don't be afraid to revisit your narrative, revise it, and share it anew, each time revealing a deeper layer of your authentic self.

Note: Sharing your story can be an emotional experience. Be mindful of your own emotional well-being and seek support if necessary. Remember, it's okay to take your time, share only what feels comfortable, and prioritize your self-care throughout the process.

Unknown Fact: Studies have shown that sharing one's personal story can lead to increased emotional well-being, stronger social connections, and even a greater sense of purpose in life. So, step into the light, dear reader. Find your voice, share your story, and witness the transformative power of human connection that unfolds before you. Remember, you are not a solitary thread in the tapestry of life; you are a vibrant hue, woven into the intricate fabric of shared experiences. Let your courage inspire, your vulnerability connect, and your authenticity pave the way for a world where stories not only entertain but heal, empower, and remind us of the profound beauty of being human.

Beyond Words: Expanding Your Storytelling Palette

While the written word holds immense power, the art of sharing your story takes many forms. Here are some ways to tap into your creative expression and paint your narrative with a vibrant palette beyond the realm of words:

- Through the Lens: Photography can capture the essence of a moment, a journey, or an emotion in a single frame. Share your story through pictures, showcasing significant landscapes, candid moments, or even symbolic objects that evoke memories and feelings. Let your lens become a silent storyteller, weaving a visual narrative that complements your written words.

- Melody and Verse: Is your voice yearning to be heard? Craft a song, write a poem, or even rap your story! Music and poetry possess the unique ability to evoke emotions and tap into the depths of our being. Let your journey find rhythm and rhyme, resonating with others on a level that transcends language.

- Brushstrokes of Expression: Art serves as a universal language, speaking to the soul through colors, textures, and form. Pick up a paintbrush, sculpt with clay, or channel your emotions onto canvas. Let your creative spirit dance on the blank canvas, translating your experiences into visual metaphors that speak volumes.

- Movement and Storytelling: Our bodies can be powerful storytellers. Consider dance, theater, or even movement-based therapies to express your journey through physical expression. Through graceful movements, powerful gestures, and silent narratives, your body can become a conduit for emotions, conveying experiences that words may struggle to articulate.

- Building with Threads: Textiles and fibers hold stories within their very essence. Consider quilting, embroidery, or even weaving to create a tangible representation of your journey. Each stitch, each knot, becomes a chapter in your narrative, culminating in a vibrant tapestry that speaks of resilience, growth, and the beauty of the human experience.

Remember, there is no one right way to share your story. Embrace your unique voice, explore different channels of expression, and let your creativity dance. As you delve deeper into your narrative, you might discover hidden strengths, uncover unexpected connections, and even embark on new creative journeys.

So, dear reader, go forth and paint your story with the vibrant colors of your being. Whether through words, images, music, movement, or any other creative avenue, share your light with the world and witness the transformative power of connection that unfolds as your tapestry intertwines with others, weaving a richer, more vibrant fabric of shared humanity. Remember, your story matters. It is a gift, a beacon of hope, and a testament to the unyielding spirit that resides within each of us. Share it with courage, share it with vulnerability, and watch as your voice lights up the world, one thread at a time.

Chapter 18: Making Fitness and Healthy Eating a Family Affair

Involving Family in Meal Planning and Cooking

Involving your family in meal planning and cooking isn't just about sharing chores – it's an opportunity to create lasting memories, build healthy habits together, and bond over delicious home-cooked meals. Turning mealtimes into a collaborative effort can be fun, rewarding, and a powerful tool for instilling positive food choices in your children and loved ones. Here are some tips to get you started:

Making Meal Planning a Family Project:

- Brainstorming Sessions: Gather everyone around the table (or even have a picnic!) and brainstorm meal ideas for the week. Let everyone voice their preferences, considering dietary restrictions and allergies. Use cookbooks, recipe websites, or even past family favorites for inspiration.

- Theme Nights: Add a touch of fun by assigning theme nights, like "Taco Tuesdays" or "Meatless Mondays." This encourages exploration of new cuisines and keeps mealtimes exciting.

- Shopping Adventures: Take the kids grocery shopping to involve them in choosing healthy ingredients. Teach them about reading food labels, identifying nutritious options, and comparing prices. Let them pick out a new fruit or vegetable to try each week.

- Recipe Research: Assign tasks like researching recipes online or trying out a new family cookbook. Older children can learn basic cooking techniques like chopping vegetables or measuring ingredients.

Turning Cooking into a Team Effort:

- Divide and Conquer: Break down recipes into smaller tasks based on everyone's abilities. Younger children can stir ingredients, set timers, or wash fruits and vegetables. Older children can help with chopping, mixing, and even grilling or using the oven under adult supervision.

- Make it Messy (and Fun): Don't be afraid of a little mess! Let kids experiment with dough, toss salads, or decorate plates with creative food art. Remember, the focus is on having fun and enjoying the process, not about achieving culinary perfection.

- Kitchen Dance Party: Put on some music and turn cooking into a family dance party! Crank up the tunes while prepping ingredients, washing dishes, or even waiting for food to cook. This adds energy and makes the whole experience more enjoyable.

- Set the Table: Encourage everyone to help set the table, lay out utensils, and light candles for a special family dinner. This builds anticipation and creates a warm, inviting atmosphere.

Bonus Tips:

- Meal Prep Together: Dedicate a weekend afternoon to prepping ingredients for the week. This saves time during busy weekdays and makes it easier to throw together healthy meals.

- Grow Your Own Food: Start a small kitchen herb garden or even a windowsill vegetable patch. Let kids water the plants and witness the process of food growing firsthand.

- Cooking Shows and Challenges: Watch cooking shows together and try out recipes you see. Organize friendly cooking competitions with fun prizes to inspire creativity and healthy competition.

- Food Safety First: Teach children basic food safety practices like handwashing, proper storage, and cooking temperatures. This ensures everyone enjoys safe and healthy meals.

Note: Remember, be patient and flexible. There will be days when things get messy, or kids lose interest. Don't force it if someone isn't feeling up to helping. The goal is to build positive associations with food and cooking, not create stress or pressure. Celebrate small successes and focus on the fun of being together as a family.

Unknown Fact: Studies have shown that families who cook and eat together regularly tend to have healthier diets, closer relationships, and better communication skills. This shared experience fosters a sense of connection and belonging, while also promoting healthier eating habits that can last a lifetime.

By involving your family in meal planning and cooking, you're not just preparing food – you're planting the seeds for a healthier future and creating memories that will nourish your family for years to come. So get in the kitchen together, roll up your sleeves, and have some fun!

Encouraging Active Play and Outdoor Activities Together

Beyond Screens and Couch Potatoes: Cultivating a Family of Adventure through Active Play and the Great Outdoors

In a world dominated by digital screens and indoor comforts, the call to adventure beckons louder than ever, especially for the tiny explorers roaming our homes. But for many families, the lure of Netflix marathons and video games often outshines the promise of muddy knees and windswept smiles. Yet, nestled within the embrace of nature and the thrill of active play lies a treasure trove of benefits for every member of the family – physical health, mental well-being, and the forging of unforgettable bonds that weather any storm. So, ditch the remotes, dust off your hiking boots, and prepare to unleash the wild hearts within, for it's time to cultivate a family of adventure through active play and the great outdoors!

Why does embracing active play and outdoor adventures hold the key to unlocking a winning family experience? Let's explore the hidden gems:

- A Playground Bigger than any Screen: From towering trees as jungle gyms to babbling brooks as musical runways, nature offers a boundless playground that ignites imaginations and challenges young minds and bodies. Climbing, skipping stones, building forts, chasing butterflies – every moment is an adventure, fueling creativity, problem-solving skills, and a connection to the world beyond the confines of four walls.

- Building Bodies and Building Memories: Active play is not just fun; it's a natural fitness program disguised as epic quests and playful sprints. From chasing siblings in the park to conquering hiking trails, families create shared memories while strengthening muscles, boosting cardiovascular health, and fostering a lifelong love of movement.

- Mending the Mind-Body Connection: Nature has a magical way of quieting the chatter of everyday anxieties. Swapping cityscapes for scenic views, inhaling fresh air, and feeling the sun on your skin works wonders for reducing stress, improving mood, and promoting a sense of peace and well-being. This holistic benefit extends to children, helping them manage emotions and find calm amidst the whirlwind of childhood.

- Strengthening Family Bonds: Shared adventures forge memories that become the glue that binds families together. From epic water balloon fights to conquering challenging hikes, families laugh, sweat, and support each other, creating a unique language of shared experiences and deeper connections. These bonds built in the face of muddy challenges and triumphant victories stand strong against the winds of life.

- Unveiling the Unexpected: Nature holds the power to surprise and inspire. Whether it's discovering a hidden pond teeming with tadpoles, witnessing a breathtaking sunset paint the sky with fiery hues, or simply noticing the intricate detail of a spiderweb, every moment outdoors offers a chance to learn, connect with the natural world, and cultivate a sense of wonder that transcends the digital realm.

Crafting Your Family's Outdoor Expedition:

- Start Small, Dream Big: Don't be intimidated by epic backpacking trips. Begin with simple excursions in your local park, a backyard scavenger hunt, or even a walk around the block. As confidence grows, graduate to bigger adventures, exploring nearby forests, hiking trails, or even planning weekend camping trips. The key is to find activities that spark joy and a sense of discovery in everyone.

- Embrace Playful Chaos: Forget rigid schedules and structured activities. Let play unfold organically, fueled by curiosity and exploration. Build forts out of fallen branches, chase fireflies in the twilight, or organize a family obstacle course through the backyard. Laughter and spontaneity are the cornerstones of successful outdoor adventures.

- Gear Up for Fun, Not Fashion: Ditch the fancy athletic wear and embrace comfort and practicality. Durable clothes, sturdy shoes, and a sense of fun are all you need to conquer the great outdoors. Remember, scraped knees and muddy clothes are badges of honor, not fashion faux pas.

- Leave the Screens Behind: This one's crucial! Let technology take a backseat. Pack binoculars instead of tablets, sing songs instead of streaming music, and create stories inspired by the world around you instead of the one on your screen. The unplugged connection with nature and each other is the true treasure hunt you're seeking.

- Make it a Learning Adventure: Turn every outing into a learning opportunity. Identify birdsong, collect colorful leaves, track animal footprints, or learn about constellations under the starry sky. The outdoors is a living classroom, brimming with fascinating lessons waiting to be discovered.

Bonus Tip: Encourage your children to take the lead! Let them choose the destination, plan the activities, and even pack the snacks. This sense of ownership fosters initiative, confidence, and a deeper connection to the outdoor experience.

Note: Remember, safety is paramount. Be aware of weather conditions, local wildlife, and potential hazards. Start with familiar environments and gradually build your comfort level and knowledge as you explore further afield.

Unknown Fact: Studies have shown that spending time outdoors reduces stress, improves cognitive function, and boosts the immune system. So, step out of the comfort zone of your digital routines and embrace the exhilarating chaos of active play and outdoor adventures with your family. Witness the spark in your children's eyes as they climb their first mountain, the joyful shouts echoing through the trees. Feel the warmth of your partner's hand as you navigate a challenging trail together, laughing at the inevitable slips and stumbles. Let the shared experiences under the vast expanse of the sky weave a tapestry of memories that will outlast any trending hashtag or fleeting video game.

Beyond the Trails: Expanding Your Outdoor Play Palette

While parks and hiking trails are the gateways to your family's outdoor adventures, the journey doesn't stop there. The world is your playground; so, explore diverse landscapes and activities to keep the adrenaline pumping and the fun flowing:

- Seek Thrills on Two Wheels: Embark on family cycling adventures, exploring winding country roads or conquering paved bike paths. The wind in your hair, the feeling of effortless glide, and the scenic landscapes whizzing by create an unforgettable shared experience.

- Embrace the Water Warriors: Whether it's splashing in a babbling brook, building sandcastles on the beach, or kayaking down a gentle river, water holds an irresistible allure for children (and adults!). Embrace the playful chaos of water fights, the thrilling coolness of a refreshing dip, and the joy of discovering hidden aquatic creatures.

- Stargazing Adventures: As twilight descends, spread a blanket under the open sky and embark on a celestial journey. Download stargazing apps, identify constellations, and marvel at the awe-inspiring vastness of the universe. This cosmic connection fosters a sense of wonder and reminds us of our place in the grand scheme of things.

- Snow Sports for Frozen Fun: If you live in a winter wonderland, embrace the frosty landscape! Build snowmen, have epic snowball fights, or conquer the slopes together, mastering the art of skiing or snowboarding. Laughter, rosy cheeks, and shared adrenaline rushes create memories that will thaw even the coldest hearts.

- Volunteer and Connect: Make your outdoor adventures meaningful by volunteering in local parks, planting trees, or cleaning up a nearby beach. These activities instill a sense of responsibility for the environment, foster community spirit, and create opportunities for families to connect with their local ecosystems.

Remember, the key is to keep it fun, keep it active, and keep it together. As you build a family that thrives on the great outdoors, you'll witness the blossoming of resilience, confidence, and a deep connection to the natural world in your children. You'll rediscover the simple joy of laughter shared under the open sky, the thrill of overcoming challenges together, and the unwavering strength of family bonds forged in the crucible of adventure. So, lace up your boots, pack your picnic baskets, and prepare to write the next chapter of your family story in the boundless pages of the great outdoors. The world is waiting, and your adventures are just beginning!

Setting a Healthy Example: Positive Influence on Loved Ones

The Ripple Effect: Setting a Healthy Example and Inspiring Lasting Change in Your Family

In the ever-expanding universe of family life, health often takes a backseat to the whirlwind of daily routines and competing priorities. Yet, nestled within the chaos lies a powerful opportunity – the chance to set a positive example and ignite a ripple effect of healthy habits that resonates through every member of your family. Remember, children, like impressionable seedlings, absorb the behaviors and attitudes nurtured around them. By adopting a proactive approach to your own health, you become the gardener, sowing the seeds of healthy choices that can blossom into lifelong well-being for your loved ones.

Why does setting a healthy example hold the key to unlocking a transformative experience for your family? Let's unpack the fertile soil of this influence:

- Leading by Doing, Not Just Saying: Children are astute observers, learning more from your actions than your words. Seeing you prioritize healthy meals, lace up your sneakers for a run, or choose water over sugary drinks sends a powerful message. Consistency and genuine enthusiasm speak volumes, far louder than lectures or empty threats.

- Breaking Unhealthy Cycles: Unhealthy habits often run deep in families, becoming unspoken traditions passed down through generations. By making conscious choices to break free from sugary snacks, sedentary evenings, and emotional eating, you rewrite the narrative. You become the agent of change, paving the way for a healthier future not just for yourself, but for your children as well.

- Fostering a Culture of Wellness: When healthy choices are woven into the fabric of everyday life, they become less like restrictions and more like natural rhythms. Family walks replace Netflix marathons, picnics with fresh fruit replace processed fast food, and bedtime stories are punctuated by deep breaths instead of endless screen time. This culture of wellness permeates every aspect of your life, creating a supportive environment where healthy habits take root and flourish.

- Building Confidence and Resilience: Seeing you navigate challenges and make healthy choices, even when it's hard, empowers your children. They learn that setbacks are temporary, that self-care is vital, and that resilience is the key to overcoming obstacles. This newfound confidence spills over into all areas of their lives, equipping them with the tools to make healthy choices independently.

- Strengthening Family Bonds: Shared activities, from cooking healthy meals to exploring new hiking trails, create shared experiences and memories. You laugh together over burnt omelets, cheer each other on during family fitness challenges, and celebrate small victories in healthy choices. These shared moments not only solidify family bonds but also forge a sense of teamwork and mutual support in the pursuit of well-being.

Planting the Seeds of a Healthy Family Tree:

- Embrace Incremental Change: Don't overwhelm yourself or your family with drastic transformations. Start small, introducing one healthy habit at a time. Swap soda for sparkling water, add a veggie into your regular meals, or replace evening TV time with a family walk. Small, consistent changes become stepping stones, leading to sustainable, long-term habits.

- Get Everyone Involved: Make it a family affair! Involve your children in meal planning, choosing fruits at the grocery store, or creating fun fitness challenges together. When everyone feels ownership of the process, motivation soars, and healthy choices become a collaborative adventure.

- Celebrate the Journey, Not Just the Destination: Don't fixate on achieving "perfection." Focus on celebrating progress, no matter how small. Applaud the extra serving of vegetables at dinner, cheer on your partner's commitment to daily walks, and offer encouragement when setbacks occur. Remember, every positive step, even a wobbly one, leads closer to your goal.

- Make it Fun, Not a Chore: Injecting playful energy into healthy choices keeps the motivation brimming. Turn grocery shopping into a scavenger hunt for colorful fruits, transform exercise into a family dance party, or create silly names for different vegetables. When learning and growth are laced with laughter, engagement skyrockets.

- Lead with Openness and Vulnerability: Show your children that healthy choices are not about rigid restrictions but about self-care and well-being. Share your own struggles, your moments of weakness, and your triumphs over unhealthy habits. This vulnerability not only strengthens your connection but also demonstrates that a healthy life is a journey, not a destination.

Bonus Tip: Don't be afraid to ask for help! Seek guidance from nutritionists, fitness instructors, or family therapists to design an approach that resonates with your unique family dynamic.

Note: Remember, change takes time, and setbacks are inevitable. Be patient with yourself and your family, offer unwavering support, and celebrate every step along the way.

Unknown Fact: Studies have shown that parents who set a healthy example are more likely to have children who adopt healthy habits, leading to improved physical and mental well-being in the entire family. So,

So, embrace your role as the gardener of your family's health.

Creating Family Fitness Traditions: Shared Experiences and lasting Bonds

Beyond Biceps and Broccoli: Weaving Family Fitness Traditions for Lasting Connection and Vibrant Well-being

In the bustling tapestry of family life, the threads of activity and healthy eating often fray under the pressures of daily routines and competing priorities. Yet, nestled within the chaos lies a potent tool for weaving stronger bonds, igniting laughter, and building a shared foundation for lifelong well-being – the vibrant fabric of family fitness traditions. These are not simply routines or checkboxes on a to-do list; they are threads of joy, woven into the tapestry of your family's story, creating memories that linger long after the sweat dries and the muscles recover.

Why do family fitness traditions hold the key to unlocking a transformative experience for your loved ones? Let's unravel the hidden gems woven into this vibrant fabric:

- Beyond Gyms and Grocery Lists: Family fitness traditions transcend the confines of sterile gyms and monotonous meal plans. They ignite imaginations, transforming exercise into playful adventures and healthy eating into culinary expeditions. Picture backyard scavenger hunts disguised as obstacle courses, family dance parties fueled by healthy smoothies, or bedtime stories punctuated by silly yoga poses. The possibilities are as endless as your creativity.

- Building Bonds that Weather Any Storm: Shared experiences through fitness forge unshakeable connections. You laugh together over clumsy yoga poses, cheer each other on during family bike rides, and celebrate the triumph of conquering a challenging hike as a team. These shared moments weave invisible threads of trust, support, and encouragement, creating a family that stands strong, not just physically, but also emotionally.

- Cultivating Champions of Movement: Family fitness traditions are breeding grounds for healthy habits. Children who grow up with movement and activity woven into the fabric of their lives develop a natural love for exercise, a confidence in their bodies, and a resilience that propels them through life's challenges. They become champions of movement, not just in the physical realm, but also in their approach to challenges and their pursuit of well-being.

- Creating Memories that Outlast Trends: As trends come and go, the laughter shared during a family water balloon fight or the thrill of conquering a climbing wall together remain etched in the tapestry of your shared story. These are the memories that become family currency, passed down through generations, reminding everyone of the joy found in movement, connection, and a healthy life.

- Inspiring Beyond the Family Circle: Your commitment to family fitness can become a beacon of inspiration for others. Witnessing your joyful adventures and shared dedication to well-being may ignite a spark in your friends, neighbors, and even extended family, encouraging them to weave their own threads of movement and healthy habits into their family narratives.

Weaving Your Family's Fitness Tapestry:

- Embrace Playfulness: Ditch the rigid routines and structured workouts. Let play be your guide! Turn exercise into a game, invent goofy workout challenges, and dance to silly music. Laughter is the most potent ingredient in the recipe for lasting memories and sustainable habits.

- Find Your Family's Groove: Explore different activities until you discover what resonates with everyone. Whether it's geocaching adventures, neighborhood bike rides, or backyard badminton tournaments, find activities that spark joy and get everyone moving, regardless of age or fitness level.

- Make it a Collaborative Adventure: Involve everyone in planning and choosing activities. Let your children contribute ideas, pick music for your family workout jams, or even take turns leading simple stretches or warm-up routines. Ownership fosters engagement and commitment.

- Celebrate Every Step: Don't get fixated on achieving perfection. Celebrate every triumph, big or small. Applaud the extra serving of vegetables at dinner, cheer on your partner's commitment to daily walks, and offer hugs and high-fives when family fitness challenges are conquered. Every step towards well-being deserves recognition.

- Focus on the Journey, Not the Destination: Remember, it's not about achieving Olympic-level fitness or competing with anyone but yourselves. Enjoy the process, the shared moments, and the laughter along the way. The joy of movement and the connection forged through shared experiences are the true treasures of family fitness traditions.

Bonus Tip: Don't be afraid to get messy! Roll in the grass during park picnics, splash each other during water balloon fights, and embrace the occasional muddy knees and windswept hair. These are the badges of honor earned in the joyful pursuit of family fitness.

Note: Remember, everyone has different fitness levels and abilities. Be inclusive, flexible, and adjust activities to accommodate everyone's needs and capabilities. The goal is to have fun, move together, and create shared memories, not to win medals or set records.

Unknown Fact: Studies have shown that families engaged in regular physical activity together experience improved physical and mental health, stronger family bonds, and a higher likelihood of maintaining healthy habits throughout their lives. So,

So, take a deep breath, lace up your sneakers, and grab your loved ones by the hand. It's time to embark on a vibrant adventure, weaving your family's unique tapestry of fitness traditions. Remember, this isn't a race against the clock or a competition for the fittest family on the block. It's a journey of love, laughter, and shared experiences that build resilience, cultivate well-being, and forge bonds that weather any storm.

Beyond the Backyard: Expanding Your Fitness Fabric

While backyard games and family dance parties are potent threads in your tapestry, the possibilities for shared adventures stretch far beyond your own four walls. Here are some ways to expand your family's fitness horizons and weave even more vibrant memories into your story:

- Embracing the Great Outdoors: Turn nature into your playground! Explore hiking trails, have epic snowball fights in the winter, or rent kayaks and conquer a gentle river together. The fresh air, stunning scenery, and sense of adventure inherent in outdoor activities will invigorate your spirits and leave you brimming with shared stories.

- Testing Your Mettle (with a Smile): Challenge yourselves as a family! Sign up for a local 5k run together, tackle a climbing wall as a team, or test your balance with a family yoga session in the park. Stepping outside your comfort zones, supporting each other through challenges, and celebrating triumphs together will build confidence and strengthen your family's spirit.

- Discovering New Horizons: Travel can be a powerful tool for forging fitness bonds. Explore new cities on foot, bike your way through picturesque landscapes, or try your hand at surfing lessons on a tropical beach. Immersing yourselves in new cultures and activities not only broadens your perspectives but also creates unforgettable memories and shared stories.

- Serving Your Community through Movement: Blend fitness with philanthropy by participating in charity walks, volunteering at soup kitchens, or organizing neighborhood clean-up events. Giving back to your community fosters a sense of purpose, teaches valuable lessons about compassion, and gets everyone moving towards a common goal.

- Turning Everyday Moments into Active Rituals: Don't let the ordinary become mundane. Turn everyday activities into playful movement adventures. Dance your way to the grocery store, have family yoga stretches before bedtime, or turn household chores into a fitness game with squats while folding laundry or lunges while sweeping the floor.

Remember, the beauty of family fitness traditions lies in their inherent flexibility and adaptability. Embrace the seasons, explore new activities, and let your creativity guide you. The most important ingredient is the joy of movement shared with your loved ones. As you weave these threads of activity and adventure into your family's story, you'll witness a powerful transformation. Your bodies will become stronger, your minds will clearer, and your bonds will deepen, creating a vibrant tapestry of well-being that resonates through generations.

So, step out of the routines, lace up your smiles, and embark on the joyful adventure of creating family fitness traditions. Let your laughter echo through the parks, your sweat mingle under the open sky, and your memories sparkle brighter than any trophy. Together, you'll weave a legacy of health, connection, and a love for life that endures, reminding everyone that the greatest prize is not a finish line, but the vibrant tapestry of experiences shared with the ones you love.

Chapter 19: Traveling with Fitness and Healthy Eating in Mind

Staying Active on Vacation: Walking, Hiking, Local Fitness Classes

Chapter 19: Traveling with Fitness and Healthy Eating in Mind

Ah, travel! The thrill of exploration, the beauty of new landscapes, the deliciousness of unfamiliar cuisines... and the potential derailment of your hard-earned fitness and healthy eating habits. Fear not, wanderlust-stricken wellness warrior! With a little planning and some clever choices, you can enjoy your adventures while keeping your body and mind happy and energized.

Staying Active on Vacation:

- Walking is your ultimate travel companion: Embrace your inner explorer and lace up your shoes. Whether it's strolling through charming cobbled streets, meandering along a sun-drenched beach, or navigating bustling city markets, walking is a fantastic way to stay active, soak in the scenery, and burn some calories. Bonus tip: Use a pedometer or step-tracking app to make it a game and challenge yourself to reach a daily goal.

- Hike for breathtaking views and heart-pumping workouts: Craving a more rugged adventure? Lace up your hiking boots and hit the trails! Hiking offers stunning vistas, fresh air, and a satisfying physical challenge. Choose trails that match your fitness level and be sure to pack ample water and sun protection. Note: Research local hiking regulations and wildlife warnings before venturing out.

- Embrace local fitness classes: Immerse yourself in the culture while getting your sweat on! Participating in a yoga class on a secluded beach, a Zumba session in a vibrant plaza, or a tai chi routine in a serene park can be a unique and memorable experience. Don't be afraid to step outside your comfort zone – you might discover a new favorite activity! Unknown fact: Many local community centers and resorts offer free or low-cost fitness classes, so be sure to inquire.

- Turn everyday activities into movement opportunities: Take the stairs instead of the elevator, explore a new neighborhood by bike, or join a guided kayak tour. Every little bit counts! Bonus tip: Pack a lightweight jump rope or resistance bands for a quick workout in your hotel room or on the beach.

Maintaining Healthy Eating Habits:

- Plan and research: Before you embark on your journey, spend some time researching healthy dining options at your destination. Look for restaurants with a focus on fresh, local ingredients, and don't be afraid to ask for recommendations from locals.

- Embrace the market: Immerse yourself in the colorful bounty of local farmers' markets. Stock up on fresh fruits, vegetables, nuts, and whole grains for healthy snacks and meals you can prepare in your hotel room or apartment. Bonus tip: Learning a few basic phrases in the local language can help you navigate the market and communicate your dietary preferences.

- Pack wisely: Fill your suitcase with travel-friendly healthy snacks like dried fruit, trail mix, dark chocolate, and protein bars. These will keep you going during long travel days and help you resist unhealthy temptations.

- Portion control is key: Even while on vacation, be mindful of your portion sizes. Opt for smaller plates, share dishes with friends, and savor each bite. Remember, you can always go back for more if you're still hungry later.

- Hydration is vital: Pack a reusable water bottle and keep yourself hydrated throughout the day, especially in hot climates. Proper hydration is essential for maintaining energy levels and preventing fatigue during your active adventures.

Remember:

- Balance is key: Don't be afraid to indulge in the occasional local treat or dessert. Enjoying new culinary experiences is part of the travel adventure! Just balance it out with plenty of healthy choices throughout the day.

- Listen to your body: Don't push yourself too hard, especially if you're not used to an active vacation. Take rest days when needed and prioritize sleep. A well-rested body is a healthy and happy body!

- Make it fun: Choose activities you genuinely enjoy. Whether it's a morning jog on the beach, a leisurely bike ride through the countryside, or a lively dance class, the key is to associate movement with pleasure.

Traveling with fitness and healthy eating in mind can be an enriching and rewarding experience. Embrace the opportunity to explore new landscapes, cultures, and cuisines, all while taking care of your body and mind. Remember, consistency is key, so even small efforts along the way will make a big difference in your overall well-being and enjoyment of your travels. Bon voyage, and happy adventuring!

Healthy Food Choices While Traveling: Planning and Research

Chapter 19: Traveling with Fitness and Healthy Eating in Mind

Ah, travel! The thrill of exploration, the beauty of new landscapes, the deliciousness of unfamiliar cuisines... and the potential derailment of your hard-earned fitness and healthy eating habits. Fear not, wanderlust-stricken wellness warrior! With a little planning and some clever choices, you can enjoy your adventures while keeping your body and mind happy and energized.

Healthy Food Choices While Traveling: Planning and Research

Maintaining a healthy diet while traveling can be challenging, but it's certainly not impossible. By planning ahead and doing your research, you can set yourself up for success and avoid unhealthy pitfalls. Here are some key strategies to keep your taste buds happy and your waistline in check:

1. Know your destination: Familiarize yourself with the local cuisine and dietary patterns before you embark on your journey. This will help you make informed choices when it comes to selecting restaurants and navigating grocery stores.

- Research regional specialties: Look for dishes that utilize fresh, local ingredients and traditional cooking methods. These are often healthier options than tourist-oriented fare.

- Understand cultural dining norms: Are portions typically large or small? Is it customary to share plates? Knowing these details can help you avoid overeating.

- Learn some basic phrases: Being able to ask for specific dietary needs or ingredients in the local language can be incredibly helpful, especially in non-English speaking countries.

2. Be a savvy planner: Don't rely on chance encounters for your meals. Take some time before your trip to research healthy dining options at your destination. Resources like:

- Travel blogs and websites: Many travel blogs focus on healthy eating and offer recommendations for restaurants and markets.

- Restaurant review platforms: Look for reviews that mention healthy options or specific dietary needs.

- Mobile apps: Apps like HappyCow and VegOut can help you find vegetarian and vegan restaurants around the world.

3. Embrace the market: Local farmers' markets are a treasure trove of fresh, seasonal produce. Stock up on fruits, vegetables, nuts, and whole grains for healthy snacks and meals you can prepare in your hotel room or apartment.

- Bonus tip: Pack reusable grocery bags to avoid plastic waste and make carrying your market finds easier.

- Note: Be aware of local food safety concerns and wash all produce thoroughly before consuming it.

4. Pack wisely: Fill your suitcase with travel-friendly healthy snacks like dried fruit, trail mix, dark chocolate, and protein bars. These will keep you going during long travel days and help you resist unhealthy temptations on the go.

- Unknown fact: Packing a small jar of nut butter and a loaf of whole-wheat bread can turn an apple or banana into a surprisingly satisfying and nutritious meal.

5. Befriend your hotel kitchen: If your accommodation has a kitchenette, make use of it! You can prepare simple, healthy meals using fresh ingredients from the market or local grocery store. This is a great way to save money and avoid unhealthy restaurant fare.

6. Don't be afraid to ask: Many restaurants are willing to accommodate dietary restrictions with a little advance notice. Don't be shy about asking for modifications to menu items or requesting healthier cooking methods.

7. Embrace portion control: Even while on vacation, be mindful of your portion sizes. Opt for smaller plates, share dishes with friends, and savor each bite. Remember, you can always go back for more if you're still hungry later.

8. Hydration is vital: Pack a reusable water bottle and keep yourself hydrated throughout the day, especially in hot climates. Proper hydration is essential for maintaining energy levels and preventing fatigue during your active adventures.

9. Make it fun: Explore the local culinary scene with an open mind and a sense of adventure. Trying new foods can be a rewarding experience, and you might just discover a new favorite dish!

10. Remember, balance is key: Don't be afraid to indulge in the occasional local treat or dessert. Enjoying new culinary experiences is part of the travel adventure! Just balance it out with plenty of healthy choices throughout the day.

Bonus Tip: Download a language learning app before your trip and learn some basic phrases related to food and dietary needs. This can be a fun and useful way to communicate with locals and ensure you get the healthy options you desire.

By following these tips and doing your research, you can make healthy food choices a priority while traveling. Remember, a little planning goes a long way in ensuring you have a happy, healthy, and delicious journey!

So pack your bags, lace up your walking shoes, and get ready to explore the world with a healthy body and a curious mind. Bon voyage!

Discovering New Cuisines: Expanding Your Palate with Moderation

Beyond Backpacks and Boulevards: Embracing Culinary Adventures with a Mindful Palate

Travel unlocks a treasure trove of experiences – breathtaking landscapes, vibrant cultures, and, of course, a tantalizing world of diverse cuisines. Each bite of a new dish unveils a story, a tradition, a unique expression of a place and its people. But amidst the whirlwind of sightseeing and souvenir shopping, the temptation to indulge in every culinary delight can arise, potentially eclipsing the mindful approach to health and well-being we strive for at home. So, how do we navigate the delectable maze of foreign flavors, savoring the cultural tapestry woven through food while maintaining a harmonious balance with our fitness and healthy eating goals?

Why does embracing new cuisines with a mindful palate hold the key to unlocking a transformative travel experience? Let's unpack the hidden spices in this flavorful adventure:

- Expanding Your Culinary Horizons: Travel becomes a sensory feast, not just for the eyes but also for the taste buds. Each new bite offers a glimpse into a different culture, its history, and its connection with the land. Embracing local ingredients and traditional dishes broadens your culinary perspectives, creating a deeper understanding and appreciation for the places you visit.

- Fueling Your Explorations: Food is the fuel that propels your adventures. Choosing balanced meals keeps your energy levels high, allowing you to conquer scenic hikes, explore bustling markets, and lose yourself in museum wanderings without succumbing to pre-flight-style crash hunger.

- A Bridge to Cultural Connection: Sharing meals with locals is a gateway to meaningful connections. Trying local specialties shows respect for their traditions, creating opportunities for conversations, laughter, and shared experiences that transcend any language barrier.

- Mindful Moderation: Unlocking the True Essence of Flavor: When we approach food with mindfulness, savoring each bite without succumbing to mindless indulgences, we truly appreciate the intricate flavors and nuances of each dish. We discover that enjoying local delicacies doesn't require overindulgence, but rather an intentional focus on quality over quantity.

- Sustainable Indulgences: Travel allows for occasional moments of culinary abandon, without jeopardizing your overall health goals. Savor that rich pastry without guilt, knowing you've balanced it with nutritious meals and active exploration throughout your trip. Remember, sustainable well-being isn't about rigid restrictions, but about making conscious choices and enjoying the occasional treat mindfully.

Bon Appétit with Balance: Savoring Your Culinary Journey

- Be a Culinary Detective: Research local specialties before you travel. Seek out dishes made with fresh, seasonal ingredients and traditional cooking methods. Ask locals for recommendations, venture beyond tourist traps, and discover hidden gems where authentic flavors reign supreme.

- Embrace Small Plates and Shared Feasts: Opt for small plates and shared meals instead of hefty portions. This allows you to try a variety of dishes without overeating, fostering a spirit of communal dining and encouraging mindful savoring.

- Make Breakfast Your Fuel Stop: Don't underestimate the power of a nutritious breakfast. Start your day with fresh fruits, yogurt, or local staples to fuel your explorations and avoid unhealthy snacking in the late morning.

- Hydration is Key: Water is your travel companion in good health. Stay hydrated throughout the day to combat fatigue, boost energy levels, and make mindful choices at mealtimes.

- Listen to Your Body: Ditch the guilt and ditch the rigid rules. Pay attention to your body's hunger cues and stop eating when you're comfortably satisfied. Remember, the goal is to enjoy the experience, not adhere to an impossible standard of perfection.

Bonus Tip: Pack healthy snacks like nuts, fruits, and granola bars for those moments when temptation lurks around the corner. Having healthy options readily available empowers you to make mindful choices in any situation.

Note: Don't be afraid to ask questions! Inquire about ingredients, cooking methods, and local delicacies. Embrace the cultural exchange and learn from the culinary wisdom of the people you meet.

Unknown Fact: Studies have shown that experiencing and understanding diverse cuisines can lead to healthier dietary choices overall, encouraging increased consumption of fruits, vegetables, and whole grains, even after returning home. So,

So, pack your sense of adventure, your curiosity, and your willingness to step outside your comfort zone. Embrace the cultural tapestry woven through food, savoring each bite with a mindful palate. Remember, mindful exploration, not culinary restrictions, is the key to unlocking a transformative travel experience that nourishes your body, soul, and connection to the world around you. As you navigate the bustling markets, climb ancient ruins, and lose yourself in the rhythm of foreign conversations, let your taste buds tell a story of cultural appreciation, mindful indulgence, and a deepened understanding of the places you call temporary home. Bon appétit, fellow adventurers!

Making Travel Part of Your Healthy Lifestyle: Active Adventures and Well-Being

Beyond Guidebooks and Getaways: Weaving Movement into Your Travel Tapestry for Vibrant Well-being

Travel promises escapes from the mundane, immersing us in breathtaking landscapes and vibrant cultures. Yet, amidst the allure of sightseeing and souvenir shopping, the temptation to relegate fitness to the realm of "once I'm back home" can whisper seductively. But why confine well-being to the familiar ground when the world itself can be your playground? Here's how to transform travel into an extension of your active lifestyle, weaving movement into your adventures for a tapestry of vibrant well-being that transcends souvenir photos and echoes long after you return home.

Why does making travel an active adventure hold the key to unlocking a transformative experience? Let's unpack the hidden treasures tucked within this adventurous pursuit:

- Beyond Tourist Trails: Fitness as Your Compass: Ditch the rigid itineraries and discover hidden gems through the lens of movement. Hike rugged mountain trails to unveil breathtaking vistas, cycle through quaint villages to connect with locals, or kayak pristine waters to witness nature's silent orchestra. Active exploration not only fuels your body, but also opens doors to authentic experiences and perspectives.

- Empowering Exploration: Fueling Your Adventures: When your body feels strong and energized, the world becomes your oyster. Conquering challenging hikes, navigating vibrant streets on foot, or dancing the night away at local festivals – embracing activity on your travels unlocks a boundless sense of possibility, allowing you to explore further, deeper, and with genuine gusto.

- Building a Bridge to Nature: Movement becomes a potent language, connecting you to the diverse landscapes you encounter. Whether it's the rhythmic pounding of your feet on a dusty desert trail, the cool caress of wind against your skin on a bike ride, or the deep breaths drawn in during a sunrise yoga session by the ocean –

active exploration fosters a profound connection with the natural world, leaving you rejuvenated and awe-inspired.

- Mindful Movement, Meaningful Memories: When you turn movement into a mindful practice, travel becomes a meditation in motion. Each step, pedal stroke, or yoga pose becomes an opportunity to connect with your body, savor the surroundings, and create conscious memories that linger long after your tan fades.

- Sustainable Well-being, Beyond Boundaries: Weaving mindful movement into your travel tapestry doesn't require regimented workouts or Olympic aspirations. It's about finding playful ways to stay active, incorporate natural movement into your explorations, and return home energized, not depleted. Remember, sustainable well-being thrives on joy, balance, and a playful spirit.

Adventure Awaits: Weaving Activity into Your Travel Tapestry

- Unleash Your Inner Explorer: Embrace diverse forms of movement! Hike scenic trails, rent bikes for city explorations, join local dance classes, or take surfing lessons. Each new activity unveils a different facet of your destination, leaving you with a kaleidoscope of unforgettable experiences.

- Seek Local Inspiration: Immerse yourself in the movement traditions of the places you visit. Take a tai chi class in China, master the samba steps in Rio, or join a morning yoga session on a serene Indian beach. Connecting with local practices broadens your horizons and creates unique cultural exchanges.

- Turn Sightseeing into Active Adventures: Ditch the crowded buses and explore your destination on foot. Walk through historic districts, navigate picturesque alleys, or climb iconic landmarks. Not only will you burn calories, but you'll discover hidden gems and connect with the city's heartbeat on a deeper level.

- Pack Playful Intentions: Remember, travel is about embracing joy and discovery. Turn walks into scavenger hunts, park picnics into frisbee matches, and impromptu dance parties in your hotel room. Injecting playfulness into your movement keeps things fun and fuels your adventurous spirit.

- Connect with Nature's Playground: Embrace the elements! Swim in waterfalls, climb trees, hike through dense forests, or simply lie under the starry sky and practice mindful breathing. Immersing yourself in nature's playground offers a unique form of movement, rejuvenating your body and spirit.

Bonus Tip: Embrace spontaneity! Don't stick to rigid plans. Get lost in winding streets, follow tempting detours, and let the spirit of adventure guide your movement. You might stumble upon hidden waterfalls, charming cafes, or breathtaking viewpoints you never knew existed.

Note: Don't compare your journey to others. This is your adventure, your pace, your body. Listen to your inner compass, choose activities that spark joy, and celebrate every step towards a vibrant, active travel experience.

Unknown Fact: Studies have shown that regular physical activity during travel not only improves physical health and mood but also enhances cognitive function, memory, and overall well-being. So,

So, step out of your comfort zone, lace up your walking shoes, and pack your adventurous spirit. Let the world be your gym, your dance floor, your yoga mat. As you weave movement into your travel tapestry, you'll discover that well-being isn't confined to familiar routines and hometowns. It becomes a passport to a vibrant life, enriching your experiences, forging deeper connections with the world around you, and leaving you with memories that shine brighter than any souvenir. Remember, travel is not just about the places you visit, but about the way you move through them. So, embrace the rhythm of your footsteps, the exhilaration of the wind in your hair, and the joyful beat of your heart as you explore. Travel with an active spirit, a curious mind, and a playful soul, and watch your well-being blossom into a vibrant tapestry that transcends destinations and endures in the echoes of your adventurous story. Bon voyage, fellow explorers, and may your journeys be filled with movement, mindfulness, and the exquisite dance of well-being in every step you take.

Chapter 20: Aging with Grace and Gratitude: Embracing Every Chapter of Your Life

Celebrating Your Accomplishments: Recognizing Progress and Milestones

Aging is a journey, not a destination. It's a tapestry woven with threads of experience, challenges conquered, and lessons learned. But amidst the inevitable wrinkles and silver strands, there's another remarkable thread running through this tapestry: the power of recognizing your accomplishments.

In the whirlwind of daily life, it's easy to let moments of triumph slip by unnoticed. The laundry gets folded, the bills get paid, the garden blooms again – just another day, right? Wrong. Each one of these seemingly mundane tasks is a milestone, a testament to your resilience, your strength, and your continued journey.

Why Celebrate? The Magic of Milestone Recognition:

Celebrating your accomplishments, big or small, isn't just about indulging in self-congratulation. It's a powerful tool that unlocks a treasure chest of benefits:

- Motivation: Recognizing your progress fuels your internal engine. Every time you acknowledge a win, your brain releases a dose of dopamine, the feel-good hormone, urging you forward with renewed enthusiasm.

- Confidence: Celebrating milestones reinforces your belief in yourself. It whispers, "You did it! You are capable of achieving great things." This newfound confidence becomes armor against self-doubt and propels you to tackle bigger challenges.

- Gratitude: Taking time to appreciate your journey cultivates an attitude of gratitude. You begin to see the beauty in the everyday, the value in perseverance, and the joy in simply being. This grateful heart adds layers of richness to your life experiences.

- Inspiration: When you celebrate your wins, you inspire others. Your jubilant spirit becomes contagious, encouraging those around you to embrace their own journeys and celebrate their triumphs.

Beyond the Trophy Shelf: Different Ways to Celebrate Your Wins:

The world of celebration is your oyster. There's no one-size-fits-all approach, so discover what resonates with you:

- Indulge in a Small Pleasure: Treat yourself to a relaxing massage, a delicious meal, or a book you've been dying to read. These little tokens of appreciation nourish your soul and remind you of your worth.

- Share Your Joy: Let your loved ones know about your accomplishment. Share your story, relive the experience, and bask in the warmth of their congratulations. Connecting with others deepens your joy and strengthens your support system.

- Document Your Journey: Keep a journal, create a scrapbook, or simply take photos to mark your milestones. These tangible reminders allow you to revisit your achievements and draw strength from them in times of doubt.

- Give Back: Celebrate your success by helping others. Volunteer your time, donate to a cause you care about, or simply offer a helping hand to someone in need. Spreading kindness amplifies your joy and creates a ripple effect of positivity.

- Set New Goals: Recognizing your progress is a springboard to even greater heights. Use your accomplishment as a launchpad to set new goals, stretching your comfort zone and embracing the exhilarating potential of the future.

Bonus Tip: Create a "Celebrations Jar." Throughout the week, write down your accomplishments, big or small, on slips of paper and toss them into a jar. Once a month, have a mini-celebration and draw out a few slips to relive and celebrate your wins.

Note: Celebrating doesn't have to be extravagant. A quiet moment of self-reflection, a heartfelt "thank you" to yourself, or a simple dance of joy in your living room is enough.

Unknown Fact: Studies have shown that people who regularly celebrate their accomplishments have stronger immune systems, less stress, and even live longer!

Embrace the Journey, Every Step of the Way:

Aging isn't about waiting for the finish line. It's about savoring the dance of each step, recognizing the beauty in the ordinary, and celebrating every victory, big or small. So, dear reader, as you turn the pages of your life's story, remember this:

- Your journey is a masterpiece. Every wrinkle, every gray hair, every scar and every smile tells a tale of strength, resilience, and life lived to the fullest.

- Your accomplishments, however big or small, are worthy of celebration. Take time to acknowledge them, let them fuel your spirit, and use them as stepping stones to even greater heights.

- You are the author of your story. Celebrate the twists and turns, the moments of triumph and the lessons learned. Embrace the present, relish the future, and age with grace and gratitude, savoring every chapter of your extraordinary life.

Remember, dear reader, the world needs your joy, your resilience, and your wisdom. Keep celebrating, keep growing, and keep embracing the magnificent adventure that is life.

Recognizing your accomplishments is one thing, but actively tracking and celebrating them adds a whole new layer of fun and excitement to your journey. Here are some creative ideas to boost your milestone mania:

- The Progress Planner: Dedicate a notebook or a section of your planner to tracking your goals and celebrating your wins. Jot down your aspirations, big and small, and as you achieve them, mark them off with flourish. Decorate your pages with stickers, drawings, or quotes that inspire you.

- The Milestone Jar: Remember the "Celebrations Jar" from earlier? Take it a step further and create a "Milestone Jar" specifically for noteworthy achievements. When you conquer a big goal, write it down on a colorful piece of paper, fold it into a beautiful origami shape, and add it to the jar. Shake it up every month or quarter, draw out a milestone, and relive the journey with a mini-celebration.

- The Gratitude Board: Visualize your wins with a dedicated gratitude board. Pin up pictures, articles, or even handwritten notes that remind you of your accomplishments. This visual tapestry will serve as a daily dose of inspiration and a reminder of your incredible journey.

- The Social Shoutout: Don't be shy! Share your victories with the world (or at least your social media circle). Post a celebratory picture, write a heartfelt message about your journey, and bask in the warm glow of congratulations and encouragement from your loved ones.

- The Time Capsule Adventure: Take a page out of history and create a time capsule for your future self. Pack it with mementos, photos, and written reflections on your current milestones. Bury it (figuratively or literally) and vow to unearth it years down the line. Imagine the joy of reliving your journey with the wisdom of your future self!

Bonus Tip: Turn your celebrations into acts of kindness. For every significant accomplishment, donate to a cause you care about, volunteer your time, or simply do something nice for someone in need. Sharing your joy multiplies its impact and enriches the lives of others.

Note: Milestones don't always have to be grand achievements. Did you finally master that yoga pose? Conquer a challenging recipe? Learn a new language? Every step forward is a milestone worth celebrating.

Unknown Fact: Research suggests that celebrating with others amplifies the positive emotions associated with achievement. So, don't be afraid to share your joy and connect with your loved ones on your journey.

Embrace the Power of Now:

As you dance through the chapters of your life, remember this: the present moment is where your milestones come alive. Savor the small victories, the daily triumphs, and the quiet moments of joy. Celebrate your journey, acknowledge your progress, and let gratitude be your compass.

Embrace every wrinkle, every laugh line, and every silver strand as a testament to your beautiful, vibrant story. You are the author, the hero, and the champion of your own life. So, raise a glass (or a cup of tea, or a smile!) to yourself, dear reader, and celebrate the masterpiece that is your journey.

Remember, the world needs your light, your laughter, and your stories. Keep celebrating, keep growing, and keep aging with grace and gratitude. Now go forth, write your next chapter, and paint it with the vibrant colors of your achievements and your joy.

Finding Joy in the Simple Things: Gratitude and Appreciation

Chapter 20: Aging with Grace and Gratitude: Embracing Every Chapter of Your Life (continued)

Finding Joy in the Simple Things: Gratitude and Appreciation

As we age, our lives morph and shift, taking different shapes and hues. The whirlwind of responsibilities, daily routines, and the inevitable accumulation of 'to-do' lists can sometimes make it feel like we're missing the point, rushing past the beauty and joy right there within reach. But amidst the clamor, lies a secret treasure – the transformative power of finding joy in the simple things.

Gratitude and appreciation, far from being passive emotions, are potent tools for unlocking profound happiness and inner peace. They act as lenses, sharpening our focus on the small, everyday moments that often get overlooked. They remind us that joy isn't always found in grand achievements or exotic adventures, but often whispers in the rustle of autumn leaves, the warmth of a cup of tea, or the genuine smile of a loved one.

Why Cultivate Gratitude? The Magic of Appreciation:

Embracing gratitude and appreciation reaps a myriad of benefits that enrich our lives and color our journeys with vibrant hues:

- Happiness Boost: Gratitude unlocks a flood of positive emotions, activating the feel-good hormones in our brains. By appreciating the simple things, we cultivate a sense of contentment and joy that elevates our well-being and fosters a brighter outlook on life.

- Stress Reduction: When we shift our focus towards appreciating what we have, the grip of worry and anxiety loosens. We begin to see challenges as opportunities, and life's bumps as stepping stones, fostering a sense of inner calm and resilience.

- Strengthened Relationships: Appreciation spills over onto those around us. Expressing gratitude to our loved ones strengthens bonds, cultivates deeper connections, and fosters a sense of understanding and mutual respect.

- Living in the Present: Gratitude anchors us in the present moment. It teaches us to savor the warmth of the sun on our skin, the fragrance of a blooming flower, the melody of a bird's song – experiences that often get swallowed by the noise of our busy lives.

Beyond Thank You Notes: Practicing Gratitude in Daily Life:

Cultivating gratitude and finding joy in the simple things isn't a spectator sport. It's an active practice, woven into the tapestry of our daily lives:

- Start a Gratitude Journal: Before drifting off to sleep, jot down three things you're grateful for that day, however small. It could be the delicious cup of coffee, the laughter shared with a friend, or the quiet beauty of a sunset. Over time, this journal will become a treasure trove of joy, reminding you of the richness of your life.

- Become a "Noticer": Train your mind to be present and aware. Take a moment to truly see the raindrops glistening on leaves, the intricate patterns in a snowflake, or the delicate hues of a sunrise. These seemingly mundane moments hold unexpected beauty waiting to be discovered.

- Express Your Appreciation: Words of gratitude have magical power. Tell your loved ones how much you appreciate them, thank the barista for their friendly smile, or simply express your gratitude for the beauty that surrounds you.

- Practice Mindfulness: Mindfulness exercises like meditation or simply focusing on your breath for a few minutes can help you quiet the mind and cultivate a sense of appreciation for the present moment.

- Celebrate the Ordinary: Turn everyday tasks into mini-celebrations. Put on music while washing dishes, take a mindful walk during your lunch break, or light a candle while enjoying a leisurely bath. These intentional acts transform routines into opportunities for joy.

Bonus Tip: Create a "Gratitude Jar." Throughout the week, write down small moments of joy or things you're grateful for on slips of paper and toss them into a jar. On a rainy day or when you need a boost, draw out a slip and let the memory of that simple joy wash over you.

Note: Gratitude isn't about denying difficulties. It's about acknowledging them while choosing to focus on the good, the beautiful, and the reasons to be happy, even amidst challenges.

Unknown Fact: Studies have shown that practicing gratitude can strengthen the immune system, improve sleep quality, and even increase lifespan!

Embrace the Symphony of Life:

As we age, life becomes a symphony of moments, each one playing its unique melody. Some notes are loud and triumphant, others soft and introspective. But every note, every experience, holds the potential for joy. By cultivating gratitude and appreciation, we learn to dance with the music of life, savoring the sweetness of laughter, the comfort of silence, and the beauty of the ordinary.

Remember, dear reader, you are the conductor of your own symphony. Choose to focus on the melodies that bring you joy, the harmonies that resonate with your soul, and the rhythm of your own grateful heart.

Leaving a Legacy: Sharing Your Wisdom and Experiences

As we traverse the tapestry of life, accumulating experiences and wisdom like threads of silver and gold, a profound question emerges: What will echo beyond the final page of our story? What legacy will we leave behind?

Legacy isn't about monuments or grand gestures. It's about the ripple effect of our lives, the whispers of wisdom we share, and the love that radiates outward from our journey. It's the laughter we spark in others, the lessons we teach gently, and the inspiration we ignite in their hearts.

Why Share Your Story? The Power of Legacy:

Leaving a legacy, however small, offers a wealth of benefits for both ourselves and those around us:

- Purpose and Meaning: Sharing our wisdom and experiences imbues our lives with purpose and meaning. It reminds us that we are not isolated islands, but threads woven into the fabric of humanity, our stories influencing and enriching the lives of others.

- Connecting Generations: Age has a wealth of wisdom to offer, a treasure trove of lessons learned and stories gathered. By sharing these, we bridge the gap between generations, fostering understanding, connection, and a sense of shared history.

- Inspiring Others: Every life, ordinary or extraordinary, holds the potential to inspire. Our struggles, triumphs, and unique perspectives can offer guidance and hope to those who follow, paving the way for them to embrace their own journeys.

- Personal Growth: The act of reflecting on our experiences and articulating our wisdom deepens our self-understanding. It forces us to confront our past, embrace our present, and envision the future with clarity and purpose.

Beyond Words: Ways to Share Your Legacy:

Leaving a legacy doesn't require grand pronouncements or a published memoir. It can be woven into the very fabric of our everyday lives:

- Storytelling: Gather your loved ones and share stories from your past. Let laughter fill the air as you recount childhood adventures, life lessons learned, and the wisdom your own elders imparted to you.

- Mentorship: Offer your time and guidance to younger generations. Become a mentor, a coach, or simply a listening ear, sharing your knowledge and experiences in a way that empowers and inspires others.

- Family Traditions: Create traditions that carry your values and wisdom forward. Teach your grandchildren your favorite recipe, share family folklore around a crackling fire, or volunteer together for a cause close to your heart.

- Living by Example: The most powerful legacy is often unspoken. Your kindness, resilience, and unwavering spirit speak volumes. Lead by example, demonstrating through your actions the values you hold dear.

- Creative Expression: Unleash your creativity! Write down your stories, paint your memories, or capture your wisdom in music or poetry. These artistic expressions can become precious heirlooms, carrying your legacy beyond your lifetime.

Bonus Tip: Start a "Legacy Box." Fill it with mementos, letters, handwritten stories, and trinkets that represent your life and values. Gift it to a loved one or leave it to be discovered after your passing, allowing your legacy to live on in a tangible way.

Note: Leaving a legacy doesn't require fame or fortune. Even the smallest act of kindness, the gentlest word of wisdom, or the unwavering love you share can ripple through generations, leaving a lasting mark on the world.

Unknown Fact: Research suggests that people who feel they have a legacy to leave behind experience improved mental health, greater resilience, and a stronger sense of purpose in life.

Embrace the Power of Connection:

As we approach the final chapters of our stories, remember this: our legacy isn't built in bronze or etched in stone. It lives in the hearts we touch, the lives we influence, and the ripples of kindness we set in motion. Share your wisdom, offer your guidance, and let your life become a beacon of inspiration for those who follow. In doing so, you leave a legacy of love, connection, and enduring light, a testament to the beautiful symphony that was your life.

Remember, dear reader, you are a storyteller, a mentor, and a guiding light. Embrace the power of your experiences, share your wisdom generously, and leave a legacy that echoes through the generations, enriching the world with the melody of your unique and extraordinary life.

Living Life to the Fullest: Every Day is an Opportunity

Ah, the golden years. A phrase often tinged with the sepia tones of nostalgia, whispering of slowing down, rocking chairs, and quiet contemplation. But what if we reframed the narrative? What if, instead of seeing age as a dimming, we viewed it as a vibrant kaleidoscope, every experience a new lens, every day a fresh opportunity to embrace life to the fullest?

Living life to the fullest isn't about ticking off bucket-list adventures or chasing youthful pursuits. It's about embracing the present moment, igniting your passions, and cultivating a spirit of adventure, no matter your age or circumstances. It's about recognizing that every sunrise is a gift, every breath a privilege, and every day a blank canvas waiting to be splashed with the bold colors of your dreams.

Why Embrace the Present? The Power of Now:

Living to the fullest isn't a future destination; it's a vibrant journey. By embracing the present moment, we unlock a treasure trove of benefits:

- Heightened Joy: Focusing on the now allows us to savor the sweetness of a grandchild's laugh, the warmth of sunlight on our skin, or the beauty of a blooming flower. We move out of autopilot and truly appreciate the richness of everyday experiences.

- Reduced Stress: The present moment is free from the anxieties of the past and the worries of the future. By anchoring ourselves in now, we release the grip of stress and cultivate a sense of peace and calm.

- Openness to Possibilities: When we embrace the present, we become more receptive to unexpected joys and serendipitous encounters. Life becomes a playground of opportunities, waiting to be discovered with an open heart and a curious mind.

- Deeper Connections: We connect authentically with others when we are fully present in the moment. Our conversations become richer, our interactions more meaningful, and our relationships blossom with genuine connection.

Beyond the Comfort Zone: Igniting Your Inner Spark:

Living to the fullest doesn't require grand gestures. It's about igniting your inner spark, the flame of your passions and interests, no matter how small:

- Reconnect with Old Passions: Dust off your paintbrush, rediscover the joy of dancing, or delve back into that unfinished novel. Rekindle the flames of your past passions and allow them to illuminate your present.

- Embrace New Adventures: Step outside your comfort zone and try something new. Take a language class, join a hiking group, or volunteer for a cause you care about. Embrace the thrill of the unfamiliar and expand your horizons.

- Nurture Your Creativity: Whether it's writing poetry, gardening, or baking the perfect apple pie, creativity is a potent elixir of life. Allow your imagination to blossom and express yourself through whatever brings you joy.

- Find Inspiration in the Ordinary: The extraordinary often hides in the ordinary. Find beauty in the morning mist, joy in the rhythm of the rain, and inspiration in the faces of your loved ones. Open your eyes to the everyday magic that surrounds you.

- Connect with Nature: Immerse yourself in the restorative power of nature. Take a walk in the park, listen to the melody of birdsong, or simply breathe in the fresh air. Reconnect with the natural world and rediscover its calming and invigorating essence.

Bonus Tip: Create a "Live to the Fullest" jar. Throughout the week, write down your small goals, aspirations, and dreams for the day. At the end of the week, draw one out and commit to making it happen.

Note: Living to the fullest isn't about achieving perfection or competing with others. It's about embracing your own journey, cherishing your experiences, and celebrating the unique mosaic of your life.

Unknown Fact: Studies have shown that people who embrace life to the fullest experience greater longevity, improved mental and physical health, and a heightened sense of well-being.

Embrace the Dance of Time:

As the sands of time shift and seasons change, remember this: life is a vibrant dance, every day a new step in the rhythm of your journey. Age is not a barrier, but an invitation to embrace the present, ignite your passions, and fill your days with the vibrant colors of your dreams. So, dear reader, step onto the stage with confidence, laugh freely, dream boldly, and embrace the boundless possibilities that lie ahead. Live each day to the fullest, savor the melody of your life, and leave a legacy of joy, laughter, and the unwavering spirit of an adventurer who danced through life with grace and gratitude.

Remember, every sunrise is a fresh start, every breath a precious gift, and every day an opportunity to write a new chapter in your remarkable story. Go forth, dear reader, with a heart full of sunshine and a soul teeming with possibility. Paint your canvas with the vibrant hues of your passions, chase butterflies of wonder, and never let the fire of your spirit dim. Let your laughter echo through the canyons of time, your kindness nourish the soil of hope, and your wisdom illuminate the path for those who follow. Remember, age is not a sentence, but a symphony, and within your story lies the power to create a masterpiece. So, with a twinkle in your eye and a song in your heart, embrace the present, dance with life, and live every day to the fullest, for your journey, dear reader, is just beginning.

Your Journey to Fitness and Well-Being Starts Now: Taking the First Step

The final page has turned, the words have sung their melody, and now you stand at the precipice of your own remarkable journey. This book, a mere compass etched with suggestions and possibilities, has served its purpose. It has painted a vision of what could be, whispered of vibrant health and newfound joy, and nudged you gently towards the path of fitness and well-being. But, dear reader, the power to step onto that path resides solely within you.

Yes, there will be moments of doubt, days when the mountain ahead seems insurmountable, and evenings when the lure of the sofa whispers sweeter than the call of exercise. But remember, my friend, every journey begins with a single step. And that first step, though small, holds the transformative power of a thousand miles.

Here, at the crossroads of intention and action, I offer you this:

- A heart filled with courage: Step out of your comfort zone, embrace the unfamiliar, and let the thrill of the unknown be your fuel.

- A mind brimming with self-acceptance: Embrace your body, imperfections and all. It is your vessel, your companion, and a testament to your unique and beautiful story.

- A spirit ignited with passion: Find the spark that sets your soul alight, the activity that makes your heart sing, and let it guide your journey.

- A hand outstretched in support: You are not alone. Seek out your companions, your cheerleaders, the ones who will celebrate your victories and hold you steady on wobbly legs.

- A voice whispering encouragement: Listen to the gentle voice within, the one that applauds your efforts, not your achievements. Let it be your compass, your guide, and your unwavering source of strength.

And above all, remember this: every change, every triumph, every drop of sweat, every shared laugh along the way – these are the brushstrokes that paint the masterpiece of your well-being.

So, dear reader, close this book, let its echoes resonate within you, and take that first step. It may be a walk around the block, a stretch in the morning sun, or a healthy meal shared with loved ones. Whatever it is, let it be your declaration, your first brushstroke on the canvas of your transformed life.

This journey is yours, your song to sing, your dance to define. With each step, you weave a narrative of strength, resilience, and blooming health. You are the author, the protagonist, and the hero of your own remarkable story. So, go forth, embrace the adventure, and remember, dear reader, your journey to fitness and well-being starts now. Take that first step, and never look back.

Maintaining Motivation and Staying on Track: Consistency is Key

The ink dries on the final page, yet the story you've embarked upon has only just begun. You've navigated the twists and turns of new goals, tackled the terrain of challenging habits, and unearthed the treasures of newfound motivation. But as the initial spark of inspiration settles, a familiar question arises: "How do I keep going?" My friend, the answer lies not in fleeting moments of enthusiasm, but in the steady beat of consistency.

Think of your path to success as a winding mountain trail. The peak, your ultimate goal, beckons from afar, bathed in the golden light of achievement. But reaching it requires more than a single, exhilarating leap. It demands the quiet determination of putting one foot in front of the other, step by step, day after day. This, dear reader, is the essence of consistency.

It's not about pushing yourself to the edge every day, burning brightly and then fading into darkness. It's about finding a sustainable pace, a rhythm that weaves itself into the fabric of your life. It's about those seemingly unremarkable choices: the healthy meal over the quick fix, the early walk before the day's clamor, the swapped glass of soda for a sparkling water. These are the brushstrokes of consistency, painting a landscape of lasting change.

Remember, motivation is a fickle friend. It flits and dances, whispering sweet promises one day and leaving you adrift the next. But consistency, that's a loyal companion, walking beside you through sunshine and storm, reminding you of your purpose with every step. It's the hand that reaches out when your resolve falters, the voice that whispers encouragement when doubt creeps in.

So, don't be discouraged by the inevitable dips in enthusiasm. They are as natural as the changing seasons, a chance to rest, reflect, and refuel. Focus instead on the quiet power of consistency. Celebrate the small victories, the tiny steps that inch you closer to your goal. Track your progress, not in grand gestures, but in the daily rituals that shape your journey. Find joy in the process, in the movement of your body, the nourishment of good food, the quiet strength that builds with each consistent choice.

And remember, you are not alone. On this mountain trail, countless others are climbing too. Some run ahead, some lag behind, but the shared path binds you together. Seek their support, share your struggles, and celebrate each other's triumphs. In their companionship, find renewed strength, in their stories, fresh inspiration.

So, dear reader, as you close this book, let the echo of consistency resonate within you. Let it be your mantra, your guiding light, the steady drumbeat that drives your journey forward. Embrace the slow burn of steady progress, the quiet hum of daily discipline, and the unshakeable power of one step at a time. For it is in this unwavering rhythm that you will conquer the hills, navigate the valleys, and finally reach the peak, not with a fleeting burst of glory, but with the deep satisfaction of a journey well-traveled, a promise kept, and a life transformed, step by consistent step.

Go forth, my friend, and paint your mountain trail with the vibrant hues of consistency. May your journey be filled with quiet triumphs, unwavering resolve, and the sweet reward of a life lived on your own terms, one step at a time.

A Lifetime of Health and Happiness: Embrace the Benefits of an Active Lifestyle

As the final lines of this book fade, dear reader, a new adventure lies before you – not an adventure mapped on paper, but one etched on the canvas of your life. An adventure where movement paints your days with vibrant hues of health and happiness, where each step forward leads you to a richer, more fulfilling existence. This, my friend, is the invitation of an active lifestyle, a symphony of well-being waiting to be orchestrated by your dedication and joy.

Remember, an active lifestyle isn't a relentless pursuit of peak fitness or a competition against chiseled models on magazine covers. It's a joyous dance with your body, a celebration of its strength and resilience. It's choosing the stairs over the elevator, laughing yourself breathless during a game with loved ones, or feeling the exhilaration of a brisk walk under a canopy of stars. It's about discovering activities that ignite your soul, set your heart aflutter, and leave you buzzing with the sweet satisfaction of movement.

But the benefits of an active life extend far beyond the physical. They weave their magic into the very fabric of your being:

- A symphony of health: Your body responds to movement with a chorus of appreciation. Improved cardiovascular health, stronger bones, sharper minds, and a resilient immune system – these are the melodies played by an active lifestyle.

- A dance with happiness: Movement unleashes a symphony of feel-good chemicals in your brain, painting your days with vibrant hues of joy and boosting your mood like a potent elixir. Stress fades, anxieties loosen their grip, and a sense of calm washes over you like a gentle wave.

- A bridge to connection: Shared activities, from team sports to leisurely walks, build bridges of connection with loved ones. Laughter echoes, stories are woven, and memories are forged in the crucible of shared movement.

- A journey of self-discovery: As you explore different activities, your body becomes your compass, guiding you to hidden strengths and revealing unexpected passions. You rediscover your capabilities, push your boundaries, and embrace the thrill of being more than you ever thought possible.

- A legacy of well-being: Your active lifestyle isn't just for you; it ripples outward, inspiring those around you to embrace movement and prioritize their health. You become a beacon of well-being, a testament to the transformative power of an active life.

So, dear reader, as you turn the final page, leave behind the doubts and anxieties. Embrace the invitation of an active lifestyle with open arms. Start small, listen to your body, and savor the joy of movement in its endless forms. Celebrate your progress, be your own cheerleader, and remember, every step, every leap, every wiggle is a brushstroke on the masterpiece of your well-being.

This journey is yours, a lifelong adventure painted with the vibrant hues of movement. With every step, you weave a narrative of strength, resilience, and a life overflowing with health and happiness. You are the choreographer, the dancer, and the artist of your own remarkable story. So, put on your dancing shoes, step onto the stage of life, and embrace the transformative power of an active lifestyle. Let the music of movement guide you, the rhythm of your heart propel you, and the joy of living an active life fill your days with sunshine and laughter.

Go forth, dear reader, and paint your world with the vibrant colors of movement. May your journey be a symphony of health and happiness, a testament to the boundless potential of an active life!

You've Got This! Encouragement and Confidence for Your Success

The ink fades, the pages whisper their lullaby, and you stand at the precipice of a new reality. This book, a compass etched with possibilities, has served its purpose. It has painted a vision of what could be, ignited a spark of ambition, and whispered words of encouragement. But, dear reader, the power to turn vision into reality rests solely within you.

Yes, there will be moments of doubt, days when the mountain ahead seems insurmountable, and nights when fear clouds your vision. But remember, my friend, within you lies an unyielding power, a wellspring of strength waiting to be tapped. This is the power of your self-belief, the unwavering conviction that whispers, "You've got this."

Let it be your mantra, this simple yet potent phrase. "You've got this" to face that daunting challenge, to navigate the labyrinth of uncertainty, to silence the chorus of negativity. Let it be a shield against doubt, a fuel for your fire, a compass guiding you towards your north star.

This journey to success is yours, your path to tread, your story to write. But you are not alone. Within you resides a hidden army – your passion, your resilience, your determination, your resourcefulness. These are your unwavering allies, your loyal soldiers ever marching alongside you. Embrace their power, utilize their strengths, and watch them pave the way for your triumphs.

And remember, success isn't a singular peak, a solitary moment of glory bathed in the spotlight. It's a winding mountain trail, a symphony of small victories, a celebration of the journey itself. It's the quiet satisfaction of pushing past your comfort zone, the thrill of learning a new skill, the joy of overcoming an obstacle. These are the brushstrokes that paint the masterpiece of your success, each one a testament to your unwavering spirit.

So, dear reader, as you close this book, let the echo of "You've got this!" resonate within you. Let it be your daily affirmation, your morning mantra, your bedtime whisper. And when doubt gnaws at your resolve, when fear threatens to paralyze, repeat it with conviction, breathe it in like a potent elixir. For within those simple words lies a truth waiting to be unlocked – the truth that you are capable, empowered, and destined for success.

Go forth, then, with your head held high, your heart ablaze with passion, and your mind brimming with unwavering belief. Embrace the challenges, celebrate the victories, and never lose sight of the indomitable spirit that whispers, "You've got this." This journey is yours, and its destination is etched in the very DNA of your being. So, step onto the path, dear reader, and paint your own remarkable story of success, one confident stride at a time.